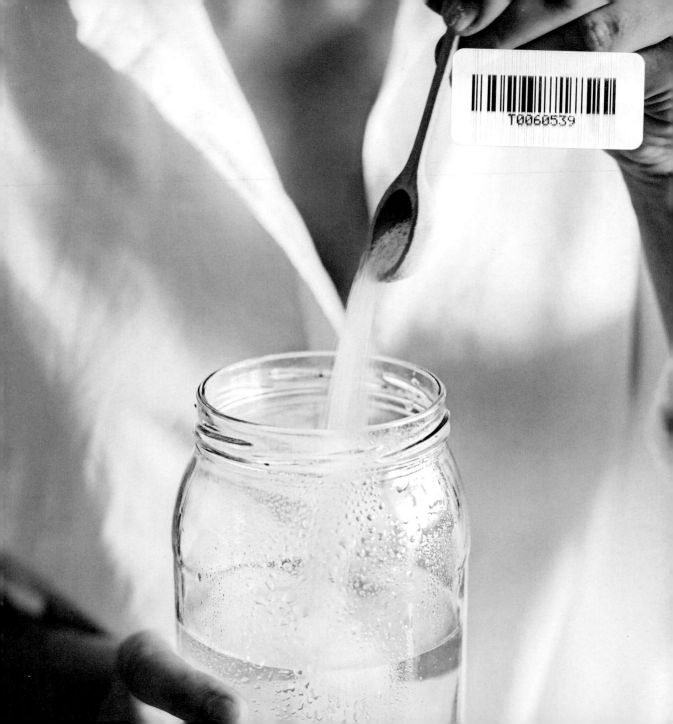

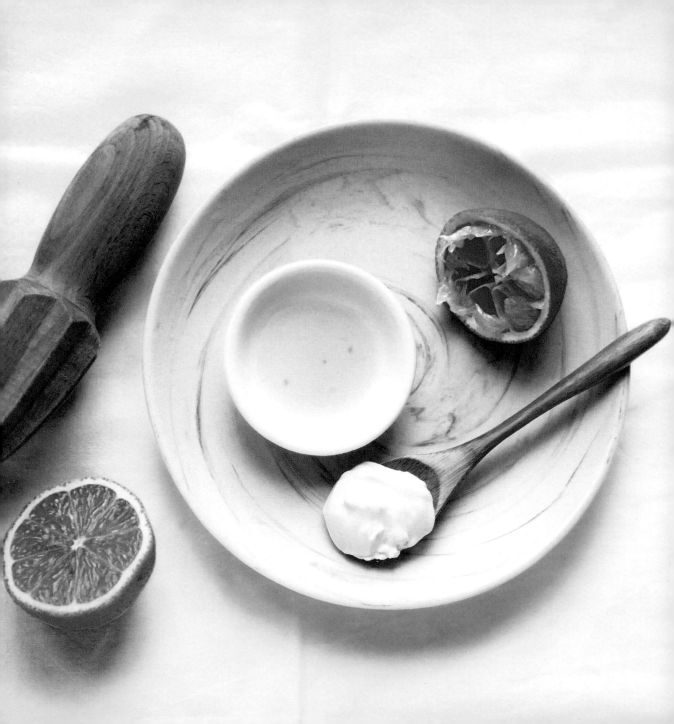

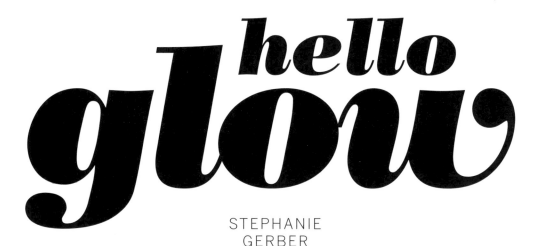

hello glow

STEPHANIE
GERBER

weldon**owen**

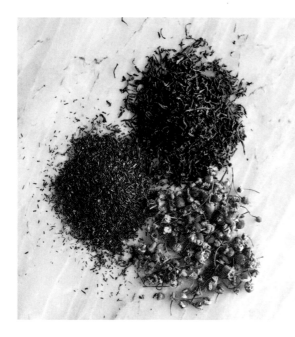
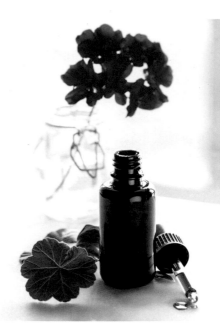

CONTENTS

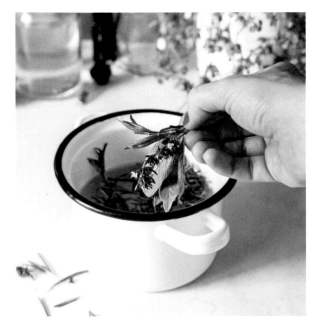
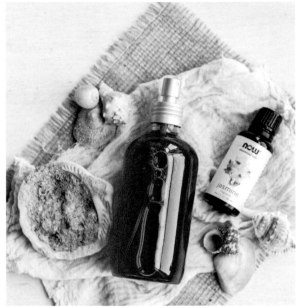

BODY

HAIR

INTRODUCTION

I GREW UP IN A FAMILY where colds were treated with a dose of garlic and echinacea, bee stings required activated charcoal, and sore throats were wrapped in wool. As a surly teenager, I was convinced my dad—who is an osteopathic doctor—was totally weird.

But along the way, a belief in those natural remedies ingrained itself. I vividly remember applying my first hair mask at age ten. My mom had serious doubts about my concoction of olive oil, mayo, and egg, but she encouraged the experimentation. My hair was greasy for a week, but I was hooked on natural beauty.

In 2011, I stumbled into blogging. I started Hello Glow to share simple projects and recipes to make myself, my life, and my home more beautiful. After having two kids, I was obsessed with all things healthy going into and on our bodies. And not only did blogging give me an excuse to try out new things, but it also helped me rediscover my sense of self after becoming a mom. Now I'm a firm believer in natural beauty and its powerful impact, inside and out.

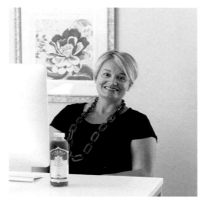

After the kids go to bed, I like to raid the fridge—for face mask ingredients! One of the best things about natural beauty is that you can get started with whatever you've got in your kitchen. (Yogurt and avocado are my go-to's for face masks, while a simple mix of coffee and olive oil is my favorite scrub.) Just don't let the do-it-yourself factor intimidate you. Keep it simple—no fancy equipment or obscure ingredients required.

Once you get over the initial "what in the world am I putting on my face?!?" freak-out, making your own natural beauty products becomes incredibly empowering. The techniques have always been simple, but somewhere along the way we forgot that all beauty products don't have to come in a package. Applying a body oil that feels and smells amazing because I made it myself feels pretty darn good.

And then there's the emotional perk of doing something nice for yourself. As a busy mom, the word "pampering" can feel awkward to me, I'll admit. But rituals like a weekly at-home facial or a regular soak in the tub with Epsom salts and coconut oil are about more than just looking good. The benefits on the inside are just as important. Whether you need to release stress or get a boost of confidence, don't feel guilty about making time for your experiments in natural beauty.

I'm so excited and proud of the simple but effective recipes in this book. I hope you delight in your natural beauty journey as much as I have. Enjoy!

Stephanie Gerber

Start Today

We're all at our most beautiful when we're healthy, so it's truly ironic that so many of today's beauty products are full of such toxic stuff. Making your own soaps, masks, scrubs, and more is a foolproof method of ensuring that only safe ingredients end up on your skin—plus, it's a great way to treat yourself to homemade spa experiences on the cheap and get that healthy glow we all crave.

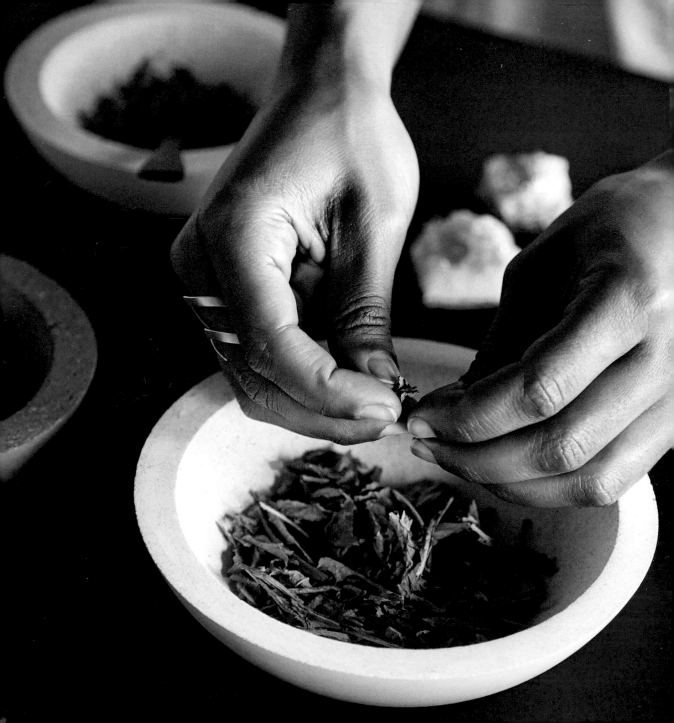

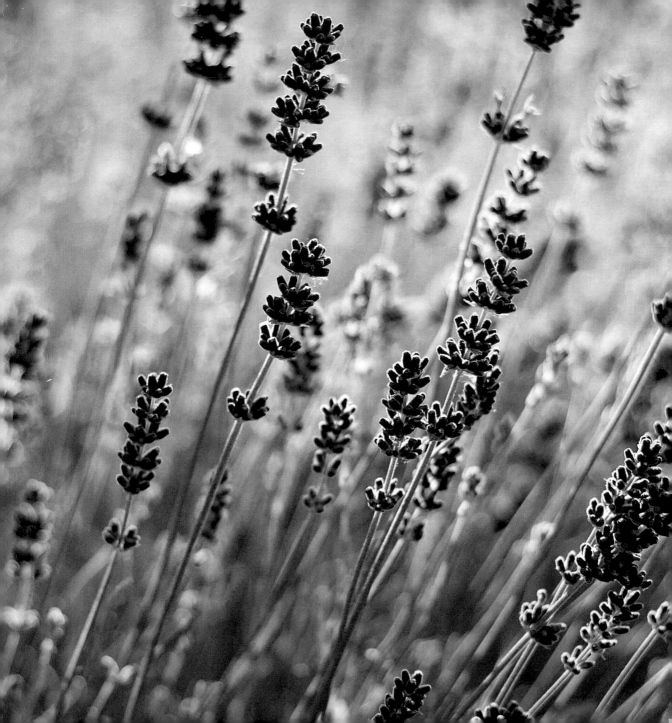

ESSENTIAL NATURAL BEAUTY INGREDIENTS

Stock up on these simple staples, and you'll be well prepared to whip up any soap, lotion, hair treatment, or skin remedy your heart desires. When you can, buy organic to avoid nasty chemicals.

Aloe Vera Known as the plant of immortality, aloe-vera gel fresh from the plant contains high levels of amino acids, minerals, and vitamins that benefit skin and hair. Reach for aloe's soothing, cooling effects when you have a sunburn, an itchy scalp, or another skin irritation. It's also effective for hydrating skin, healing acne, and lightening skin discoloration.

Apple-Cider Vinegar The main ingredient in apple-cider vinegar is acetic acid, but it contains lactic, citric, and malic acids as well. All those natural alpha hydroxy acids work together to gently exfoliate by dissolving dead cells. Applying ACV to your face also delivers beneficial enzymes, proteins, and good bacteria deeper into the skin. It's antimicrobial, antibacterial, and antiseptic, and it helps balance pH—thus it's considered a great remedy for acne, dandruff, and other skin and hair issues.

Avocado Rich in vitamins, minerals, and healthy fats, avocado and avocado oil are both deeply moisturizing for skin and hair. This fruit's omega-3 and omega-9 fatty acids hydrate and soften skin, while its plant nutrients and vitamins A, D, and E repair environmental damage.

Baking Soda Who knew that one of the most versatile natural beauty ingredients is also the least expensive? An easy cleanser for all skin types, baking soda absorbs anything it comes in contact with—and that includes excess oil and gunk in your pores. And adding baking soda to a bath can ease sunburn pain, itching, and inflammation.

Beeswax Often used to thicken beauty recipes like balms and salves, this natural bee product hydrates dry skin and creates a protective barrier to seal in all that nourishing moisture. Bonus: Beeswax also has natural antibacterial and antifungal properties.

Carrier Oils These plant-based extracts come from a nut or seed. They're ideal for moisturizing and protecting skin, and are often used to dilute essential oils.
TYPES argan, castor, coconut, grape-seed, jojoba, olive, rosehip-seed, sea buckthorn, sunflower-seed, sweet almond, tamanu

Castile Soap Castile is a plant-derived, biodegradable soap that can be used as a base for DIY beauty products, like body wash and hand soap, as well as on its own as a gentle household cleaner.

Clay Known for its ability to draw out toxins, oil, and impurities, clay also tightens and tones skin. Many are absorbent and rich in minerals, and they can jump-start circulation to reduce puffiness and large pores.
TYPES kaolin, bentonite, French green, Moroccan red

Cocoa Butter With a delicious chocolate scent, cocoa butter coats skin and protects against moisture loss. Rich in vitamin E, it helps stimulate collagen production, which can improve skin tone and help prevent stretch marks.

Dairy Your skin will love organic, whole-fat dairy products like milk, yogurt, and cream. The fats hydrate and soothe skin, the lactic acid gently cleanses and exfoliates, and the probiotics help inhibit acne outbreaks.

Essential Oils These distillations of your favorite botanicals have incredible healing and soothing properties that, when put to good use, can transform skin. That's because the molecules in essential oils are much smaller than those in most skin creams, so they can penetrate pores more deeply to nurture skin from the inside out.

Honey This natural beauty wonder is antibacterial, antifungal, and antiseptic, and its ability to heal and repair skin makes it a go-to beauty ingredient. Honey is also a natural humectant, which means it helps your skin draw in and retain moisture to keep you glowing. Try to find raw, organic honey—it's the most beneficial for facial care.

Lemon The juice from this bright citrus is an effective astringent that cuts through the oil on your skin and scalp. Its alpha hydroxy acids exfoliate, reducing the appearance of sun and age spots, as well as acne scars. Lemon juice can kick-start the cleansing of your body's lymphatic system (which helps purge waste from tissues), while lemon essential oil acts as a diuretic to reduce the appearance of cellulite.

Oats Along with fiber, oats are also packed with healthy fats and antioxidants that hydrate and rejuvenate skin. Often used in gentle cleansers, oats exfoliate dead skin, while their natural saponins create soaplike foam to draw out and absorb dirt and toxins. A natural anti-inflammatory that also balances skin's pH, oats make a soothing addition to baths when you've got irritated skin.

Salt While great for cleansing and exfoliating skin, natural sea salts can also deliver a dose of skin-loving vitamins and minerals, such as magnesium, potassium, calcium, and sodium. Epsom salt is particularly rich in magnesium sulfate, which helps your body produce energy and impacts at least 300 enzyme systems. And salt baths and scrubs allow your body to absorb these nutrients through the epidermis, as well as improve circulation and skin tone.

Shea Butter Softer than cocoa butter, shea butter has a silky texture that's easily absorbed into the skin. Its vitamins A and E help restore elasticity, relieve conditions like eczema and psoriasis, and protect from environmental damage.

Tea White, green, and black teas contain powerful antioxidants that help combat sun exposure by absorbing UV rays. And after sun exposure, tea's tannic acid and antioxidant catechins and polyphenols can reduce inflammation and help reverse the aging effects of the sun. They also make fantastic natural hair dyes and can play a soothing role in cleansers, toners, and masks.

Witch Hazel Witch hazel is a common astringent used to cleanse skin and tighten pores. Made by steaming twigs from the witch hazel shrub, the extract delivers skin-healing antioxidants—plus a cooling sensation that soothes irritated skin and calms conditions like eczema and psoriasis. Look for pure witch hazel that isn't diluted with skin-drying alcohol.

How Long Will My Recipe Last?

This is one of the most common questions—and one of the hardest to answer. Here are a few rules for getting the longest life out of your recipe.

MAKE SMALL BATCHES Most recipes only take a few minutes to mix up, so it's better to start small and remake often rather than having it spoil.

ENJOY IT FRESH Recipes with fresh ingredients should be used immediately. You can keep them in the fridge, but they probably won't last more than a week.

AVOID WATER Recipes without water, like oil-based creams and balms, will last the longest. Six months is a good estimate, as most carrier oils won't survive much longer at room temperature. If a recipe calls for water and you aren't using the product all in one go, make that water distilled!

DOSE IT WITH VITAMINS For a natural preservative, add a few capsules of vitamin E to your recipe. It contains natural antioxidants that can extend the shelf life of your products.

GO BY THE SNIFF TEST If it smells bad, get rid of it. Better safe than sorry.

STORE IT PROPERLY Keep your homemade beauty products in airtight containers in a cool, dry spot. Consider refrigerating your creations, which can extend their shelf life.

Ingredients to Avoid

Start your natural beauty journey off on the right foot by purging your cabinet of items that contain:

TRICLOSAN AND TRICLOCARBAN A common synthetic "antibacterial" chemical found in liquid and bar soaps that's been shown to impair immunity.

FORMALDEHYDE, TOLUENE, AND DIBUTYL PHTHALATE (DBP) A toxic trio found in nail polish and removers. Avoid these ingredients in personal care products as well.

FRAGRANCE Companies aren't required to disclose what's in the fragrance found in everything from deodorant to lipstick, so steer clear of these mystery chemical cocktails.

OXYBENZONE A common sunscreen ingredient that's been proven to disrupt the hormone system.

PARABENS Avoid this common preservative in shampoos, lotions, and cosmetics. If it ends with "-paraben" such as methyl-, isobutyl-, and propyl-, toss it out today—it mimics estrogen in the body and is linked to cancer.

SODIUM LAURYL SULFATE AND SODIUM LAURETH SULFATE (SLS) These surfactants are commonly found in shampoo, bubble bath, and body wash, and may cause acne.

COAL TAR HAIR DYES Dark hair dyes and shampoos often contain coal tar ingredients like aminophenol, diaminobenzene, and phenylenediamine, which are all associated with cancer.

BUTYLATED HYDROXYANISOLE (BHA) A likely carcinogen often found in lipstick and cosmetics.

HYDROQUINONE Often present in skin-lightening creams, this chemical has been connected to cancer, organ toxicity, and skin irritation.

PHTHALATES (DBP, DEHP, DEP, AND OTHERS) These scary chemicals, which are found in synthetic fragrance, nail polish, and hairspray, are known to interfere with the endocrine system.

POLYETHYLENE GLYCOL (PEGS) A major threat to the environment, these plastic microbeads are luckily on their way out. Avoid them in the meantime.

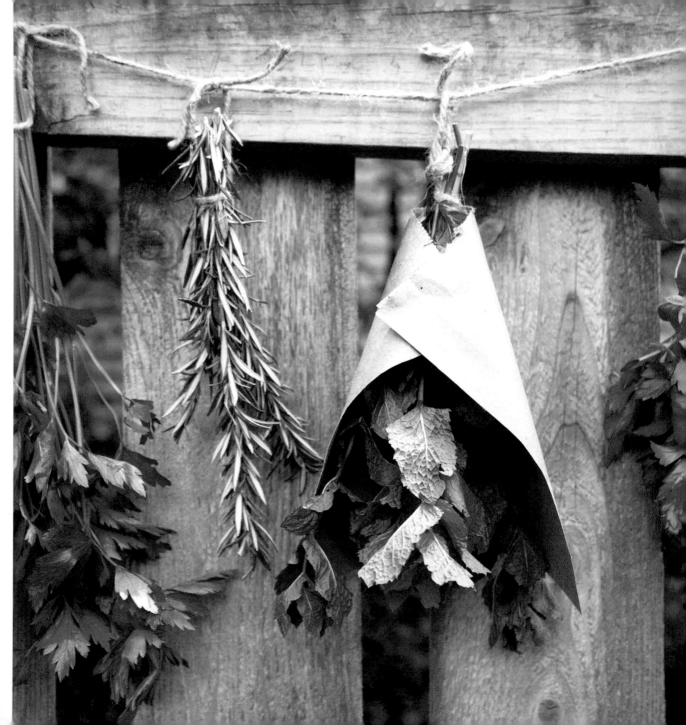

PRESERVING YOUR BOTANICALS

Stocking your window box is just as important as your pantry—fresh, aromatic herbs in your beauty recipes will make them so much more enjoyable. But no need to toss or freeze your botanicals as they expire or the weather turns chilly. Drying them is an easy way to stretch out their home-grown benefits all year.

1 / Choose a dry, warm location where your herbs can hang without disruption for up to a few weeks. This spot needs great air circulation in order to keep bacteria and mold at bay. (Avoid the kitchen, where steam can add moisture to the air.) Once you've found a good location, string up a length of twine horizontally, just like a clothesline.

2 / On harvest day, cut your herbs midmorning, after the dew evaporates but before the sun gets too high in the sky and cooks them. Remove any brown or wilted leaves, brush off dirt or bugs, and rinse with fresh water. Pat them completely dry—I mean completely! Moisture is your enemy.

3 / Bind the herbs into small bunches with 8-inch (20-cm) pieces of twine. Tie them upside down to the twine clothesline in your spot, leaving some space between each bundle.

4 / Gather some brown-paper grocery bags, enough so there's one for each bundle, and then cut each bag into a 10-by-10-inch (25-by-25-cm) square.

Roll your squares into loose cones around the herbs and secure them with tape. This covering will help keep the herbs dry and dust-free.

5 / Let time do its thing. Depending on your climate, it can take anywhere from a few days to a few weeks for your herbs to completely dry. When the leaves easily crunch between your fingers, take down the bundles, unwrap the herbs, and remove the leaves from the stems.

6 / You can store the botanicals chopped or whole. I sometimes crush them in a coffee grinder to make my own custom powders. Put them in an airtight container and use within 1 year.

Tip / You can also use those smaller brown-paper lunch sacks, if you've got some on hand. Before tying your herb bundles to the line of twine, poke a hole in the bottom of each sack. Insert the bundle into the bag and draw the twine up through the hole, then hang them up to dry.

Beauty Herb Garden

Plant and harvest these beneficial botanicals to use in face masks, hair rinses, DIY soaps, and more!

CHAMOMILE This soothing herb contains alpha-bisabolol, which improves skin's healing process and helps reduce wrinkles.

LAVENDER Not only does it smell heavenly, this beauty wonder heals skin, encourages new skin-cell growth, and boosts hair's shine.

MINT This herb grows like crazy, so you'll have lots for your face—and a few mint juleps! It's a great spot treatment because it contains pimple-clearing salicylic acid.

ROSEMARY Rosemary's astringent powers are great for oily skin. It also has antioxidants, iron, and calcium that reduce signs of aging.

SAGE Naturally anti-inflammatory and antimicrobial, sage can reduce excess oil and help with blemishes.

THYME A member of the mint family, immune-boosting thyme fights acne (sometimes better than benzoyl peroxide) and is thought to lower blood pressure as well.

WHAT'S YOUR TYPE?

Crafting your own natural beauty products gives you the freedom to customize your routine and address specific skin or hair concerns. So make it count by taking a careful look at your skin's texture, coloration, and oil/dryness ratio before you start whipping up beauty concoctions in your kitchen.

OILY

THE SIGNS Do you see large pores when you look in the mirror? Do you often have shine on your face, regardless of the temperature? These are common complaints when overactive sebaceous glands secrete too much sebum, causing oily skin. While excess oil can be a bummer as a teenager, the good news is that it can lead to fewer lines as skin ages.

THE FIX Pick a cleanser that lathers well and use weekly clay masks to remove oil and debris from deep down in the pores. And don't skip the moisturizer—overdrying the skin can actually cause oil glands to increase output! A lightweight moisturizer or serum with an oil that won't clog your pores should do the trick.

CLEANSER Foaming Honey Cleanser, page 24
TONER Balancing Rosemary-Thyme Toner, page 28
MOISTURIZER Brightening Geranium Moisturizer, page 37

COMBINATION

THE SIGNS If your skin is oily in some places and dry in others, congratulations: You're one of millions of women with the most common (and possibly the most vexing) skin type. For those with combination skin, the T-zone (the nose, forehead, and chin) is usually oily and prone to blackheads, while the cheeks feel flaky and dry.

THE FIX This skin type calls for a customized approach. A mild foam cleanser will carry away T-zone oil without overdrying other parts of the face, while an apple-cider vinegar toner won't irritate pores. It's okay to apply different moisturizers to different areas, if you can't find one that works for your whole face. During the day, go with a moisturizer that has sunscreen, but at night use something more hydrating for dry areas, like jojoba or sunflower oil.

CLEANSER Soothing Calendula + Chamomile Cleansing Grains, page 27
TONER Cucumber-Peppermint Face Mist, page 28
MOISTURIZER Camu Camu Vitamin C Serum, page 37

DRY

THE SIGNS If your pores are very small, your skin feels tight immediately after cleansing, and you find yourself prone to fine lines, then you most likely have dry skin.

THE FIX Stick with creamy or oil-based cleansers that won't strip the skin of its natural oils, and avoid harsh toners that can make skin feel tight. Serums with natural humectant ingredients like glycerin are perfect for combating the fine lines that can plague dry skin. Choose a heavier moisturizer, like a rich facial oil, to seal in hydration at night.

CLEANSER Oil-Cleansing Balm, page 24
TONER Rose + Aloe Vera Post-Workout Face Wipes, page 31
MOISTURIZER Replenishing + Age-Erasing Rosehip Lotion, page 38

A NOTE ON SENSITIVE SKIN

Your skin can be sensitive, regardless of type. This means it's especially susceptible to redness or irritation caused by certain ingredients or heat. It helps to do a patch test with new treatments.

Do a Patch Test

It's always a good idea to test products or recipes for allergic reactions before slathering them on your face—especially if they include an ingredient that you've never used before. Apply a small amount of the product to an inconspicuous spot, like the inside of your arm or leg. Wait 5 to 10 minutes to see if any redness or irritation develops, then rinse. To be extra cautious, I recommend waiting 24 hours; if you don't see or feel any adverse reaction, it's likely safe to use.

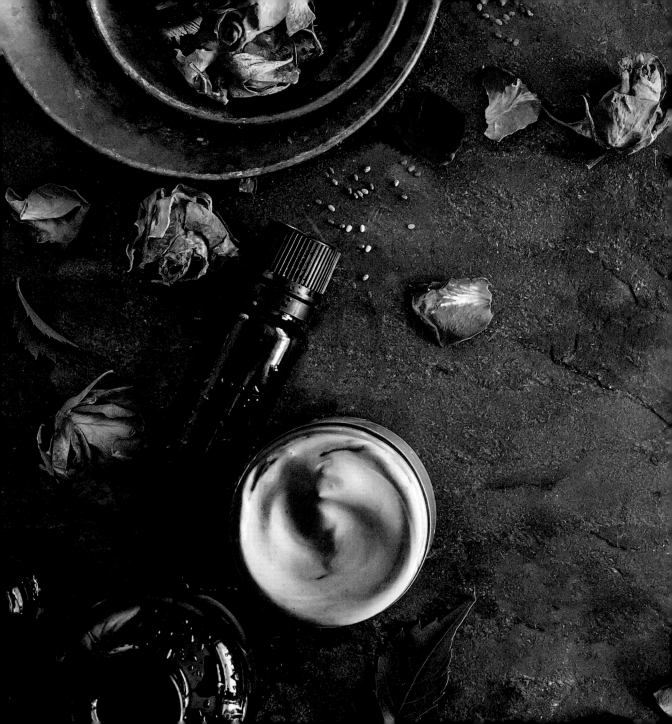

FACE

Put your best face forward
with more than 50 recipes
for cleansers, toners,
moisturizers, scrubs, serums,
masks, makeup, and more.

SKINCARE BASICS

Hello, beautiful! Yes, I mean you. While everyone has something they'd love to change about their face's texture or tone, a natural beauty regimen does more than fix your so-called problem areas. Instead, it's all about feeling comfortable in your own skin and making self-care a priority. Here's an easy-to-execute skincare regimen that will open your eyes to the benefits of regular DIY facial treatments.

DAILY

1 / Cleanse There's no better way to both start and end each day than by cleansing your face to break down and remove all traces of makeup, dirt, and sunscreen. Pick a cleanser designed for your skin type that doesn't leave your face feeling dry or tight.

2 / Tone Using a toner is not only refreshing, it also helps equalize the skin's pH after cleansing, bringing it back to its natural levels. Toners remove any leftover makeup or oily residue from cleansers too. Using a cotton ball or a spritzer, apply toner to your face after every cleansing.

3 / Apply a Serum Deliver a strong dose of concentrated nutrients to the skin with a serum. Thanks to their lightweight consistency, serums are quickly absorbed and penetrate deeper than moisturizers. Apply a few drops to clean hands and gently pat onto your face. Wait 90 seconds or longer to allow the serum to sink into the skin before moisturizing.

4 / Moisturize After applying serum, it's time to add a layer of hydrating moisturizer to soften and protect skin overnight and during your day. For daytime, you might want a lighter consistency moisturizer with SPF included. This final layer creates a protective barrier for skin—keeping in all those good ingredients you just applied and keeping out all the dirt, UV rays, and pollutants that you encounter in your day-to-day life.

5 / Mind the Eyes The eye area gets a workout throughout the day with all that smiling, squinting, and blinking. So nourish the thin skin around your eyes with a cream that hydrates and protects against aging. To use, dab a small amount on the outside corners of your eyes, being careful not to rub or tug on the fragile skin.

TWICE A WEEK

Exfoliate Exfoliation is a key part of your skincare regimen. Removing dead skin cells reveals a brighter complexion and allows your serums and moisturizers to better absorb into the epidermis. Twice a week, add grains to your cleanser or polish with a gentle face scrub after toning. Apply to the skin with your fingertips in small circular motions, avoiding the eyes.

ONCE A WEEK

Apply a Mask Treating yourself to a face mask once a week delivers nourishing antioxidants and botanicals, deep-cleans your skin, and targets specific issues, like excess oil or dryness. After toning, apply the mask to your face with clean hands and let it sit for 10 to 15 minutes, then rinse with lukewarm water.

SENSITIVE SKIN

Sensitive skin needs gentle, soothing ingredients to avoid irritation and redness. Look for products that are free of allergy-triggering preservatives and fragrances.

BOTANICALS

Calendula   Cucumber

ESSENTIAL OILS

Rose   Lavender

CARRIER OILS

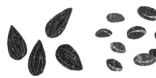

Sweet Almond   Argan

ACNE-PRONE SKIN

Acne-prone skin wants naturally purifying, astringent, and anti-inflammatory treatments. Opt for lightweight ingredients that are easily absorbed into the skin.

BOTANICALS

Witch Hazel   Peppermint

ESSENTIAL OILS

Tea Tree   Lemon

CARRIER OILS

Grape Seed   Jojoba

AGING SKIN

Call in antioxidants and natural vitamins to help heal damaged skin and improve texture, and use oils rich in fatty acids to reduce any inflammation.

BOTANICALS

Green Tea   Avocado

ESSENTIAL OILS

Neroli   Sandalwood

CARRIER OILS

Rosehip Seed   Pomegranate

Oil-Cleansing Balm

Cleansing with oil may seem kind of strange at first, but it's great for all skin—even oily faces. Why? Because oil dissolves oil, clearing out tough pore-clogging dirt while delivering beneficial oils deeper into the epidermis.

1 / Measure and mix the jojoba, grape-seed, and castor oils with the beeswax in a small heat-safe glass bowl.

2 / Boil 2 inches (5 cm) of water in a small saucepan, then lower the heat. Warm the bowl in the saucepan until the beeswax melts.

3 / Pour the mixture into the container and let cool. Add the vitamin E capsules and allow them to dissolve, then drizzle in the geranium essential and tea-tree oils with a pipette. Stir, let cool completely, and cover with the lid.

4 / At night, rub a very small amount into dry skin for 1 minute, then massage with wet hands for 30 seconds. To remove, wipe off with a damp, warm muslin cloth.

MATERIALS	TOOLS	RECOMMENDED FOR
2 tablespoons jojoba oil	Measuring spoons	Normal to dry skin
2 tablespoons grape-seed oil	Spoon	
1 tablespoon castor oil	Small heat-safe glass bowl	**FREQUENCY OF USE**
1 teaspoon beeswax	Small saucepan	1 to 2 times per week (or daily if followed by a foaming cleanser)
2 vitamin E capsules	3-ounce (90-mL) dark lidded container	
2 drops geranium essential oil	Pipette	**STORAGE ADVICE**
1 drop tea-tree oil	Muslin cloth	Use within 6 months

Foaming Honey Cleanser

A foaming cleanser is a perfect follow-up to an oil balm—it chases away lingering gunk and works far down inside those pores. Add honey's anti-inflammatory, moisture-sealing perks, and you've got a treat for all skin types.

1 / Measure and combine the honey, liquid castile soap, and distilled water in a large measuring cup. Stir gently—try to avoid making too many bubbles!—until the honey is all dissolved and combined.

2 / Stir in the avocado oil and use a pipette to add your preferred essential oil. With a funnel, transfer the mixture to a bottle with a handy pump dispenser.

3 / To use, first swirl the bottle gently until you've recombined the ingredients. Then pump a small amount of the mixture into your hand, add a little water from the tap, and massage onto your face and neck. Rinse with warm water to wash away those suds (and dirt).

MATERIALS	TOOLS	FREQUENCY OF USE
⅓ cup (120 g) honey	Measuring cups and spoons	Daily
⅓ cup (80 mL) castile soap	Spoon	
3 tablespoons distilled water	Pipette	**STORAGE ADVICE**
1 teaspoon avocado oil	Funnel	Use within 3 months
2 to 3 drops essential oil (see page 23 for the best oil for your skin type)	8-ounce (240-mL) bottle with hand pump	
	RECOMMENDED FOR	
	All skin types	

Short and Sweet

For an even simpler honey cleanser recipe, you just need one ingredient. You guessed it—honey! Fair warning, this method is a little stickier and can take a bit longer to remove, but you'll still enjoy all the benefits of a honey cleanser. Massage a small amount of the sweet stuff onto your face with your fingertips. To remove, wet a washcloth under warm water and place it over your face. Let it sit for a few seconds, then gently wipe your face to remove the honey. Repeat until all the honey is gone and your face is clean.

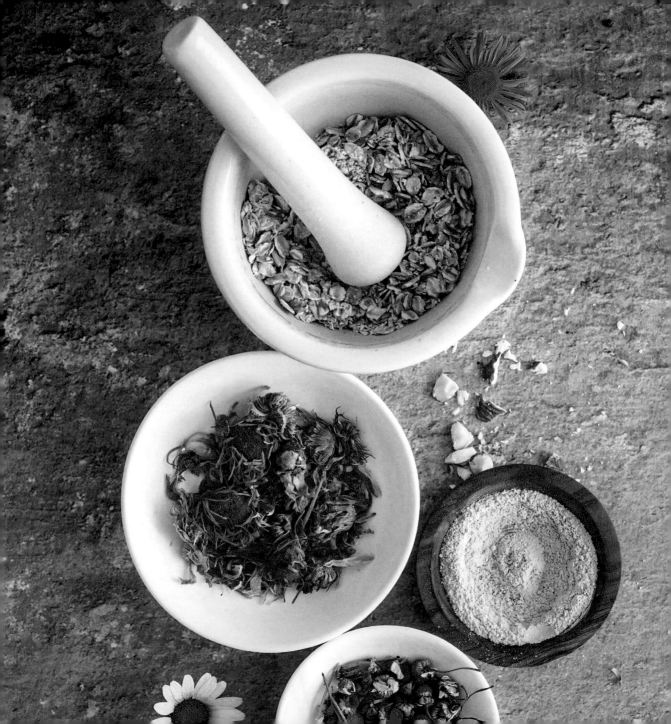

Soothing Calendula +Chamomile Cleansing Grains

This majorly effective trio of clay, oats, and dried flowers soaks up dirt and makeup, gently exfoliates, and stimulates circulation to revitalize your skin. The fine powder of cleansing grains draws out impurities—leaving your face soft, smooth, and glowing—while the herbal power of chamomile and calendula calms any redness or blemishes.

1 / Measure out the oats, almonds, chamomile, and calendula. Use a coffee grinder to crush them into fine individual powders.

2 / Combine the powders, then pour the dry mix through a fine-mesh strainer into a non-metal bowl. (Metal tools can interfere with clay, so go with plastic, wood, or ceramic.)

3 / Portion out and add the clay with a non-metal measuring spoon.

4 / Use a pipette to add the drops of chamomile essential oil and stir with a non-metal spoon to combine. Transfer to a glass jar with an airtight lid.

5 / To use, pour 1 to 2 teaspoons into the palm of your hand and mix in a tiny amount of tap water, making a paste. (You can get the skin-softening benefits of lactic acid by using milk instead of water, or opt for rose water to hydrate the skin or green tea for a dose of age-fighting antioxidants.)

6 / Use your fingertips to massage the paste into your skin, working in circular motions. Rinse with water, or leave the cleanser on your face for a few minutes to use as a nourishing mask. Follow up with toner and moisturizer.

Tip / Bacteria aren't invited to this cleansing party! To prevent spoilage, store the mixture in a dry place, and pour it into your palm or dole it out with a clean spoon at each use.

MATERIALS

¼ cup (20 g) oats

¼ cup (40 g) almonds

3 tablespoons dried chamomile flowers

3 tablespoons dried calendula flowers

½ cup (70 g) kaolin clay

10 drops chamomile essential oil

Liquid of your choosing

TOOLS

Non-metal measuring cups and spoons

Coffee grinder

Fine-mesh strainer

Non-metal bowl

Pipette

Non-metal spoon

10-ounce (300 mL) lidded glass jar

RECOMMENDED FOR

All skin types

FREQUENCY OF USE

Daily

STORAGE ADVICE

Store in a lidded jar and use within 1 year

CUSTOMIZE FOR YOUR SKIN TYPE

OILY Replace the kaolin clay with bentonite and add 1 to 2 tablespoons charcoal powder.

MATURE To erase age spots, swap the oats with ground rice. Add 2 tablespoons matcha tea powder.

SENSITIVE You can soothe redness with 1 to 2 tablespoons anti-inflammatory ingredients, such as honey powder or finely ground dried roses or lavender.

Cucumber-Peppermint Face Mist

On a hot day, nothing beats a rejuvenating spray with cooling cucumber and uplifting peppermint. Spritz it on any time you need a little extra moisture—its natural ingredients won't dry out your skin or clog your pores.

1 / Measure the distilled water and bring it to a boil in the saucepan, then remove from the heat.

2 / Add the peppermint tea bags and steep uncovered for 20 minutes. Take out the tea bags and discard.

3 / Peel and chop the cucumber. Mash through a fine-mesh strainer to extract ¼ cup (60 mL) juice.

4 / Using a funnel, pour the juice and ¼ cup (60 mL) tea into the spray bottle. Add the peppermint essential oil with a pipette, then replace the cap and shake.

5 / To use, spritz on your face after cleansing or whenever you need a quick refresher during the day.

MATERIALS	TOOLS	RECOMMENDED FOR
1 cup (240 mL) distilled water	Measuring cups and spoons	All skin types
4 peppermint tea bags	Small saucepan	
1 cucumber	Vegetable peeler	**FREQUENCY OF USE**
15 drops peppermint essential oil	Knife	As needed
	Fine-mesh strainer	
	Funnel	**STORAGE ADVICE**
	4-ounce (120-mL) spray bottle	Refrigerate and use within 7 to 10 days
	Pipette	

Balancing Rosemary-Thyme Toner

Don't skip the post-cleanse toner! It corrects pH levels, removes oily residue, and tightens skin. This toner blends the exfoliating acids of apple-cider vinegar with the zit-fighting power of thyme, rosemary, and tea-tree oil.

1 / Start by measuring the distilled water and bringing it to a boil in a small saucepan. Remove from the heat.

2 / Add the dried rosemary and thyme, and steep uncovered for 20 minutes.

3 / Filter out the herbs with a fine-mesh strainer. Transfer the liquid to the bottle using a funnel.

4 / Add the apple-cider vinegar and the tea-tree oil. Give the bottle a good shake to mix the ingredients.

5 / To use, first apply a bit to your neck to check for sensitivity. Apply to your whole face with a cotton pad after washing your face in the morning and evening.

MATERIALS	TOOLS	RECOMMENDED FOR
1 cup (240 mL) distilled water	Measuring cups and spoons	Oily or acne-prone skin
2 teaspoons dried rosemary	Small saucepan	
2 teaspoons dried thyme	Fine-mesh strainer	**FREQUENCY OF USE**
2 tablespoons apple-cider vinegar	10-ounce (300-mL) bottle	Daily
¼ teaspoon tea-tree oil	Funnel	
	Cotton face pads	**STORAGE ADVICE**
		Refrigerate and use within 7 to 10 days

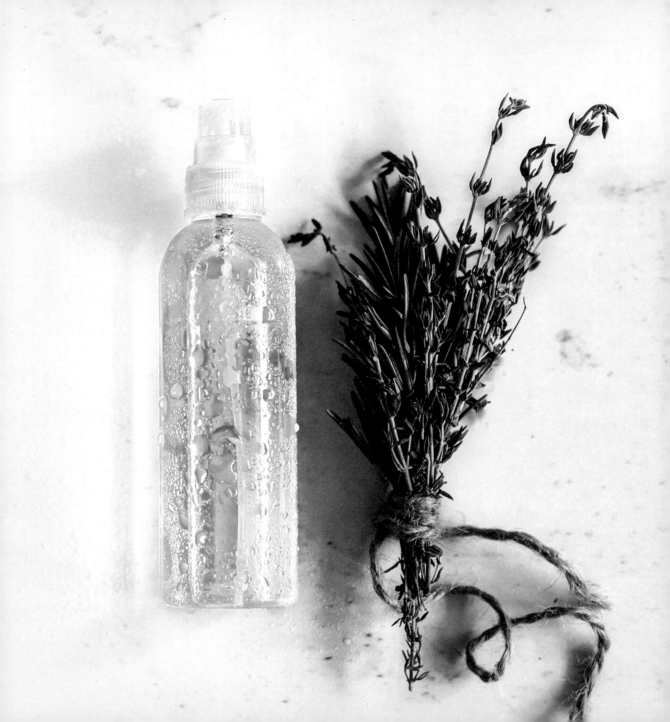

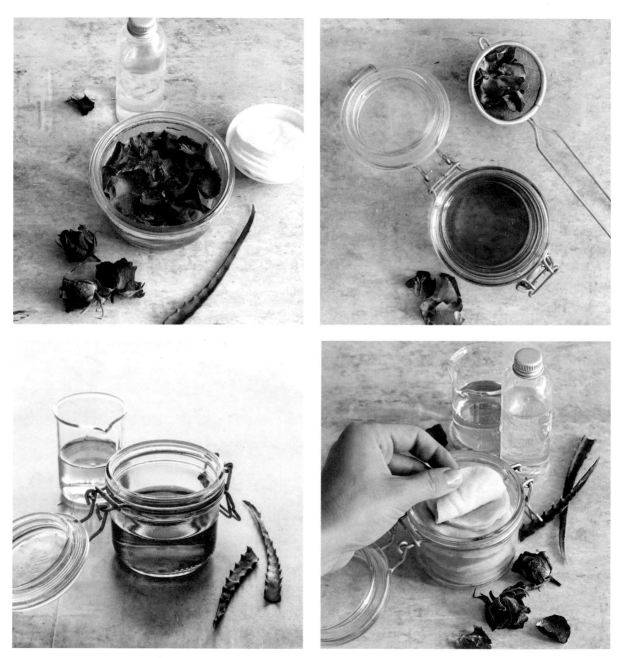

Rose+Aloe Vera Post-Workout Face Wipes

These face wipes are the perfect pick-me-up when you're short on time. Full of antioxidants, witch hazel sweeps away grime and leaves your skin feeling cool and revived. You can use them to tone skin after cleansing—or as a quick post-exercise wipe-down for your face and chest.

1 / First things first: Let's make that witch hazel more aromatic by infusing it with dried roses. Rose petals are packed with antioxidants that can calm skin irritation and help reverse signs of aging. (No roses? Try lavender, arnica, or calendula.) Place the flowers in one of the jars and pour the witch hazel over them, then replace the lid and shake thoroughly to coat the petals. The witch hazel will quickly turn a gorgeous pink color.

2 / Store the infusion in a cool, dry place and let it sit for 1 to 2 weeks. Shake the jar every other day or so.

3 / Using a fine-mesh strainer, pour the liquid into a medium bowl, filtering out and discarding the rose petals.

4 / Add the aloe-vera gel and stir together with a spoon until combined.

5 / Stack your face pads in the second jar, pressing them together tightly.

6 / Slowly pour the witch hazel–aloe vera mixture over the pads until fully saturated. Save any leftover liquid for your next batch.

7 / Replace the lid, and flip the jar over to fully disperse the liquid. Allow 1 hour for the pads to soak up all that juice!

8 / To use, pick up a pad with clean, dry fingers. Wipe over your face or other areas in need of a clean sweep.

Tip / Don't want to use pads? Then go the environmentally conscientious route: Mix ¼ cup (60 mL) infused witch hazel with 2 tablespoons aloe vera and 2 tablespoons glycerin, and transfer to a spray bottle with a funnel. Use the spray for a refreshing mist or after cleansing to hydrate and tone. Avoid your eye area.

MATERIALS

1 cup (240 mL) witch hazel

½ cup (8 g) dried rose petals

⅓ cup (80 mL) fresh aloe-vera gel

20 to 40 cotton face pads

TOOLS

Measuring cups

2 10-ounce (300-mL) wide-mouth lidded jars

Fine-mesh strainer

Medium bowl

Spoon

RECOMMENDED FOR

All skin types

FREQUENCY OF USE

Daily

STORAGE ADVICE

Use within 3 months

OTHER USES FOR WITCH HAZEL

BLACKHEAD BUSTER
Mix 1 teaspoon bentonite clay and 1 teaspoon witch hazel. Apply to the affected area. Let dry and rinse.

VARICOSE VEINS Apply witch hazel to a washcloth and hold over varicose veins to temporarily reduce swelling.

Apples

Apples contain natural alpha hydroxy acids that gently exfoliate by dissolving dead skin cells, which makes them a great ingredient for getting that healthy glow. And despite its smell, apple-cider vinegar is a rockstar natural beauty ingredient: It utilizes acids to even out skin tone and delivers beneficial vitamins, mineral salts, and amino acids deeper into the skin. These simple apple beauty recipes will nourish the face, body, and hair.

EXFOLIATING APPLESAUCE MASK

2 tablespoons sugar-free applesauce

1 tablespoon ground oats

1 teaspoon honey

2 teaspoons lemon juice

Combine the applesauce, oats, honey, and lemon juice in a small bowl. Apply the mixture to your face and neck and leave on for 10 minutes. As you wash off the mask, gently rub in circular motions to slough off dead skin cells. Towel dry and follow up with your favorite moisturizer.

GREEN TEA FACIAL TONER

1 green tea bag

¾ cup hot water

¼ cup (60 mL) apple-cider vinegar

Steep the green tea bag in the water. Let the tea cool to room temperature, then discard the tea bag and add the apple-cider vinegar. Apply the toner with a cotton ball or spritz with a spray bottle—it will combat oil without drying out your skin, and it can even help fade scars and sun spots. Store in your refrigerator for up to 10 days.

APPLE AT-HOME SKIN PEEL

1 teaspoon apple-cider vinegar

1 tablespoon sugar-free applesauce

Clean your face of all makeup, then combine the apple-cider vinegar with the applesauce and stir until well mixed. Using clean hands, apply the mask to your face, avoiding the eye area. Let sit for 10 to 15 minutes, then remove with a soft cloth and cool water. I recommend this mask at night or before a shower, as the apple-cider vinegar scent tends to linger.

SUNBURN SOOTHER

1 cup (240 mL) apple-cider vinegar

½ cup (110 g) baking soda

Did you end up a little more than sun-kissed after a day at the beach? Add some apple-cider vinegar and baking soda to your bath water to soothe that sunburn.

Other Uses for Apples

DIY DEODORANT

Apple-cider vinegar is great for neutralizing odors—including your own. Simply swipe some on your armpits to combat bacteria. (Don't worry, that telltale vinegar smell will dissipate.)

CLEANSING APPLESAUCE SCALP TREATMENT

Apply ½ cup (140 g) sugar-free applesauce directly to your scalp and hair after shampooing. The malic acid will break down any clogged hair follicles and dead skin lingering on the scalp. Let sit for 10 minutes and then rinse. Conditioner is not necessary—your locks will be left shiny and clean.

DETOX HAIR MASK

What's better for your hair than apple-cider vinegar? Apple-cider vinegar plus clay! This hair mud mask strips out chemicals, heavy metals, and synthetic product buildup from your follicles, roots, and scalp. In a medium non-metal bowl, mix ½ cup (70 g) bentonite clay with 1 cup (240 mL) distilled water and ¼ cup (60 mL) apple-cider vinegar. Add more water if needed to create a smooth consistency. Apply all over your hair and scalp, let sit for at least 30 minutes, and rinse.

Simple At-Home Facial

A facial doesn't have to cost a ton of money or include a bunch of overly complicated steps. It can be as simple as spending a few extra minutes on your skincare regimen once or twice a week to exfoliate and apply a mask. For me, watching a favorite show on Sunday night wouldn't be the same without yogurt and avocado slathered all over my face. Make facials a part of your weekly routine and you'll soon look forward to them!

1 / Prep Remove all makeup, and make sure your hands are clean. Use a headband to pull back your hair.

2 / Exfoliate Baking soda is wonderful for exfoliation—the texture is just right for a gentle scrub. Add a small amount of milk or water to the baking soda to make a paste. Then, using your fingers, massage it into your skin with small, circular motions. Start with your jaw and move upward, working the scrub into blackhead-prone areas like the chin, forehead, and nose. (Always avoid the eye area.) Rinse with warm water, and there you have it—a super-inexpensive at-home dermabrasion!

3 / Steam A hot washcloth is the perfect way to give yourself a quick steam. Estheticians know this step is the key to opening pores, increasing circulation, and prepping skin so that masks and moisturizers can easily penetrate the pores and do their thing. For this steam, simply wet a washcloth under hot water (but not too hot—don't burn yourself!), wring out excess water, and apply it to your face until the washcloth cools. Do this step two or three times.

4 / Apply a Mask It may sound simple (just one ingredient?!), but you can't go wrong with a full-fat organic Greek-yogurt facial mask once a week. (Just make sure the yogurt has no added sugar, which can accelerate aging.) Let the yogurt's lactic acid, probiotics, and fatty acids exfoliate dead skin cells, soften fine lines, and lighten age spots. Liberally apply the mask to your face and neck with clean fingers, avoiding the eye area as always. Leave the mask on for between 15 and 20 minutes, then remove gently with warm water and a washcloth.

5 / Moisturize Don't be scared of putting oil on your skin! Gently massage a small amount of coconut oil (jojoba oil would also work) over your face and neck. It's a great way to end the facial—and the smell makes you feel like you're on vacation.

MATERIALS

1 tablespoon baking soda

Milk or water

½ cup (140 g) organic, full-fat, plain Greek yogurt

1 to 2 teaspoons coconut oil

TOOLS

Measuring cups and spoons

Washcloth

RECOMMENDED FOR

All skin types

FREQUENCY OF USE

Weekly

MAKE THE MASK JUST FOR YOU

DRY SKIN
Mash and add ½ avocado and add 1 tablespoon olive oil.

ACNE-PRONE
Smash ½ banana until smooth and add 1 teaspoon turmeric.

DULL SKIN
Add 1 tablespoon each fresh lemon juice and honey.

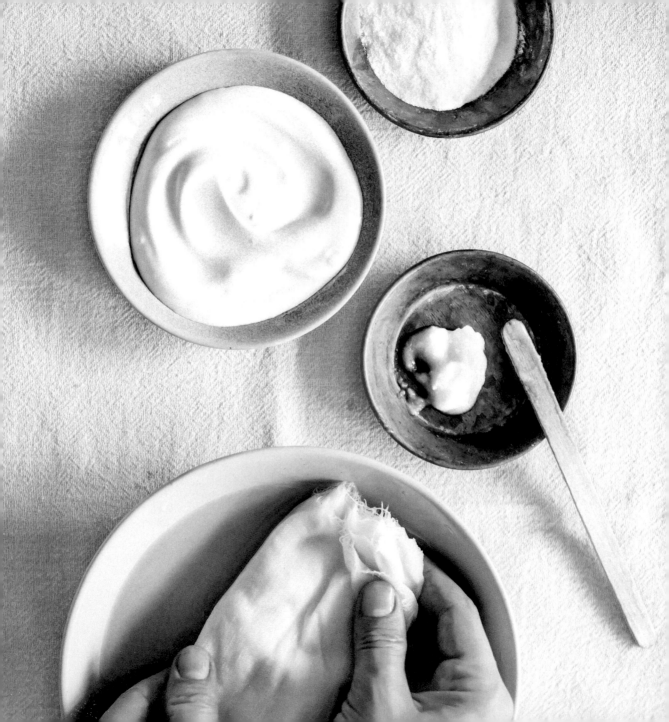

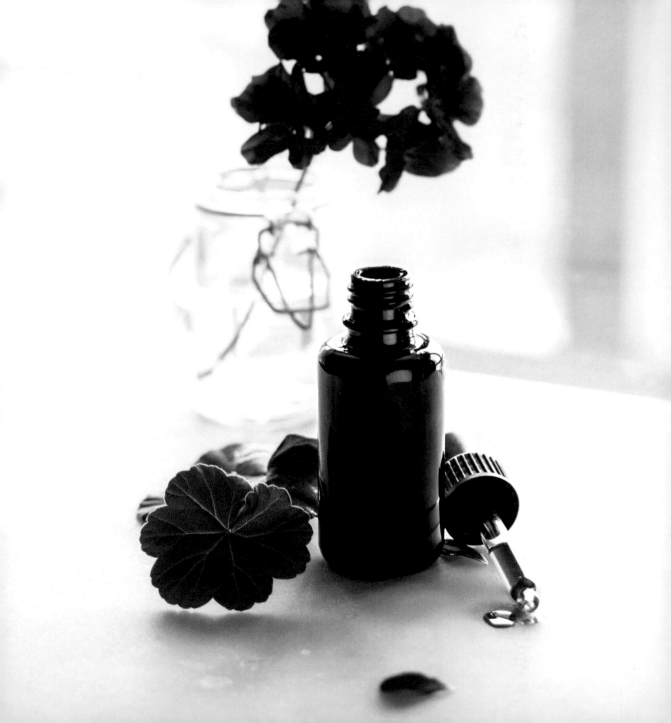

Brightening Geranium Moisturizer

Jojoba and geranium help skin regulate oil production without clogging up pores. Plus, sandalwood is a natural anti-inflammatory alternative to hydrocortisone, and lemon's vitamin C fights acne and hyperpigmentation.

1 / Using a measuring spoon and funnel, pour the jojoba and grape-seed oils into a dark glass bottle.

2 / Add the geranium, sandalwood, and lemon essential oils drop by drop with a pipette. Replace the cap and shake to combine the oils.

3 / To use, dispense 6 to 8 drops of oil into your hands and rub them together to activate the oils. Press your hands on either side of your face, then apply by pressing onto your face, neck, and chest.

MATERIALS	TOOLS	FREQUENCY OF USE
2 tablespoons jojoba oil	Measuring spoon	Daily
2 tablespoons grape-seed oil	Funnel	
18 drops geranium essential oil	4-ounce (120-mL) dark glass bottle with dropper	STORAGE ADVICE
8 drops sandalwood essential oil	Pipette	Use within 6 months
2 drops lemon essential oil	RECOMMENDED FOR	
	Normal to oily skin	

Camu Camu Vitamin C Serum

Camu camu is an antiviral, vitamin C–packed fruit from the Amazon rain forest. When combined with aloe vera and glycerin, it creates a powerful serum that fights free radicals and promotes collagen growth.

1 / Measure and then combine the camu-camu powder with the distilled water in a small bowl. Mix with a spoon.

2 / Using a funnel, pour the mixture along with the fresh aloe-vera gel and glycerin into a small dark glass bottle.

3 / Replace the cap and shake the bottle to combine the ingredients. Shake again before each use.

4 / The serum is best applied at night. Smooth a small amount over your clean face, neck, and chest. Let it absorb for at least a minute and follow with moisturizer.

MATERIALS	TOOLS	FREQUENCY OF USE
2 teaspoons camu-camu powder	Measuring spoons	Daily
1 tablespoon distilled water	Small bowl	
2 tablespoons fresh aloe-vera gel	Spoon	STORAGE ADVICE
2 tablespoons glycerin	Funnel	Use within 3 months, or refrigerate for a longer shelf life
	4-ounce (120-mL) dark glass bottle with dropper	
	RECOMMENDED FOR	
	Dry, aging, or normal skin	

Replenishing +Age-Erasing Rosehip Lotion

Loaded with vitamins and fatty acids, rosehip-seed oil is the latest go-to anti-aging remedy. Combine it with skin-nourishing jojoba and carrot-seed oils for a rich treatment that combats wrinkles and improves face texture.

1 / Boil 2 inches (5 cm) of water in a small saucepan, then turn the heat to low. Mix the jojoba oil and beeswax in a small heat-safe glass bowl. Put it in the saucepan.

2 / Let the wax melt, take the bowl off the heat, and stir in the rosehip-seed oil. Let cool to room temperature.

3 / Use a pipette to add the carrot-seed and rose absolute essential oils. Stir to combine.

4 / Pour the room-temperature rose water into a small bowl. Turn the hand mixer on low and slowly pour in the oil mixture, then blend on medium until creamy.

5 / Transfer the cream to a lidded jar. To use, apply a thin layer to your face after cleansing.

MATERIALS	TOOLS	RECOMMENDED FOR
3 tablespoons jojoba oil	Small saucepan	Normal to sensitive skin
1 tablespoon beeswax	Measuring spoons	
1 tablespoon rosehip-seed oil	Small heat-safe glass bowl	FREQUENCY OF USE
12 drops carrot-seed essential oil	Spoon	Daily
6 drops rose absolute essential oil	Pipette	
	Small bowl	STORAGE ADVICE
3 tablespoons rose water	Hand mixer	
	4-ounce (120-mL) lidded jar	Refrigerate and use within 3 months

Hibiscus Bliss Whipped Moisturizer

Here we're infusing coconut oil with hibiscus, known as the Botox plant for its skin-firming and healing properties. Whipping the oil makes for a frothy texture that goes on nice and easy—and feels heavenly on the skin.

1 / Measure out the hibiscus tea and use a coffee grinder to crush it into a fine powder.

2 / Bring 2 inches (5 cm) of water to a boil in a small saucepan. Reduce the heat to low and warm the coconut oil in a small heat-safe glass bowl in the pan.

3 / Stir in the hibiscus powder with a spoon, then cover and simmer on the lowest heat setting for 1 hour.

4 / Use cheesecloth to strain the tea out of the oil over a medium bowl. Let the oil cool until it's almost solid.

5 / Whip with a mixer on medium for 3 to 5 minutes; you'll end up with a pretty pink cream. Transfer to a lidded glass jar. Use (and enjoy!) as often as needed.

MATERIALS	TOOLS	RECOMMENDED FOR
2 tablespoons hibiscus tea	Measuring cups and spoons	Dry, aging, or normal skin
1 cup (215 g) coconut oil	Coffee grinder	
	Small saucepan	FREQUENCY OF USE
	Small heat-safe glass bowl	As needed
	Spoon	
	Cheesecloth	STORAGE ADVICE
	Medium bowl	Use within 6 months
	Hand mixer	
	8-ounce (240-mL) lidded amber glass jar	

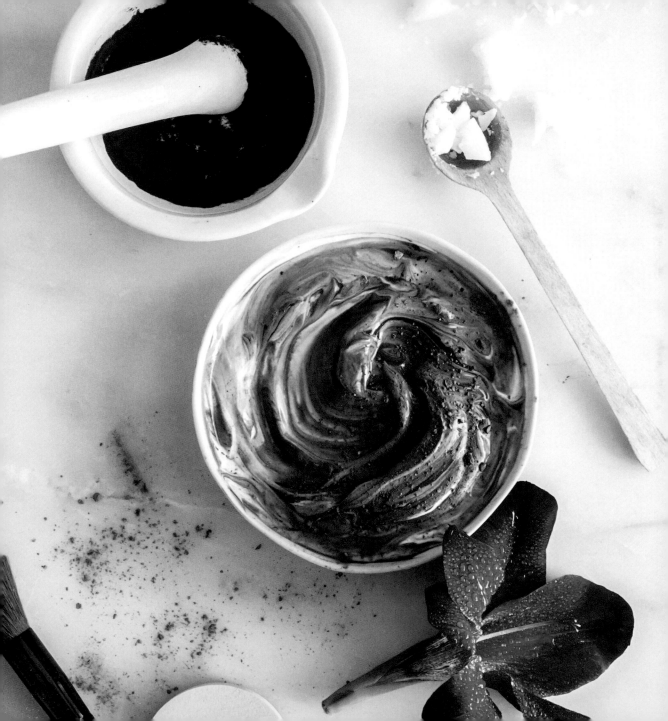

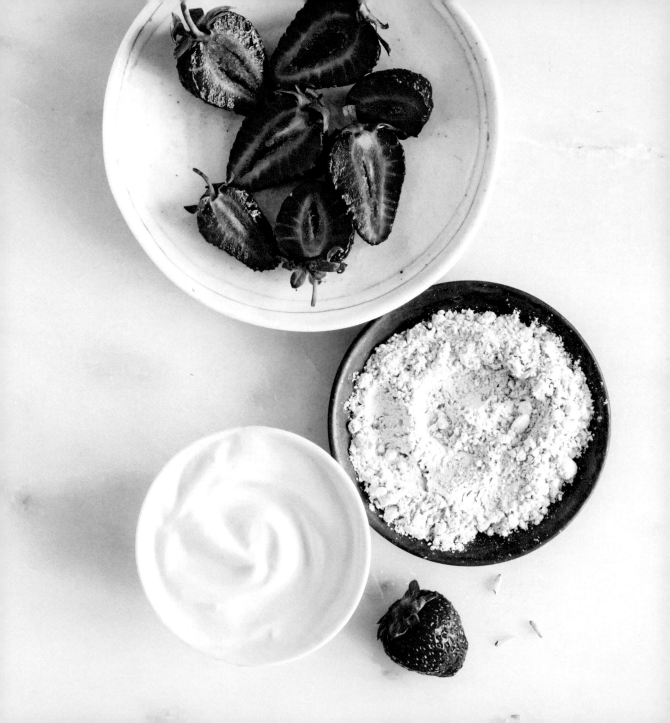

Strawberry Face Polish

Around here, we love putting strawberries on our faces almost as much as we love eating them! They're full of vitamin C—a crucial component in collagen production—and salicylic acid, which zaps dead skin cells.

1 / Crush the white rice in a coffee grinder until it's a fine powder. These grains will gently exfoliate your skin.

2 / Mash the strawberries in a small bowl with a fork.

3 / Add to the bowl the Greek yogurt, which boasts lactic acids that aid in removing the top layer of dead skin cells. Stir the mixture with a spoon to combine. When it's smooth, mix in the ground rice powder.

4 / To use, apply the polish with your fingers to a clean face. Move it in small circles around the face and neck, then let the mask sit for a few minutes to give the chemical exfoliation time to work. Rinse it off with warm water and revel in your newly smooth skin.

MATERIALS	TOOLS	FREQUENCY OF USE
2 tablespoons uncooked white rice	Coffee grinder	2 to 3 times per week
2 strawberries	Small bowl	
	Fork	
2 tablespoons organic, full-fat, plain Greek yogurt	Spoon	STORAGE ADVICE
	RECOMMENDED FOR	Refrigerate covered and use within 1 week
	Normal to oily skin	

Anti-Acne Spot Treatment

Tea-tree oil and garlic both help fight the pesky bacteria that causes breakouts, while jojoba oil soothes inflamed skin and prevents dreaded dryness. This spot treatment works best when it's fresh, so use it up right away.

1 / Cut the garlic clove in half and finely chop it, or mash it thoroughly with the back of a spoon. (You can also use a mortar and pestle, if you have one handy.)

2 / Measure the jojoba oil and add it, along with the garlic, to a small bowl. Using a pipette, drizzle in 1 to 2 drops tea-tree oil and stir to mix into a paste.

3 / To use, apply the paste to acne spots or pimples with a clean finger or Q-tip. Don't be afraid to leave pieces of garlic on pimples—it may look crazy, but they do best when they have time to work their magic.

4 / Leave the spot treatment on overnight and wash it off in the morning.

MATERIALS	TOOLS	FREQUENCY OF USE
1 clove fresh garlic	Knife or spoon (or mortar and pestle)	As needed
½ teaspoon jojoba oil	Measuring spoon	
1 to 2 drops tea-tree oil	Small bowl	STORAGE ADVICE
	Pipette	Best if used immediately
	Spoon	
	Q-tip (optional)	
	RECOMMENDED FOR	
	Normal to oily skin	

Luminous Turmeric Face Mask

Borrow a tried-and-true beauty ritual from Indian brides, who have long used turmeric in head-to-toe scrubs and face masks to brighten up their skin before their weddings. The vividly colored spice works wonders as an exfoliant and also helps tame skin inflammation. If you have sun or age spots, turmeric can reduce pigmentation and even out skin tone too.

1 / Combine the rice flour, turmeric, honey, and milk or yogurt in a small bowl, and stir with a spoon to make a paste. Feel free to add in more milk or yogurt if the mixture is too thick.

2 / Apply the mask to your face and neck with clean fingers, avoiding the eye area as always. Leave the mask on for 15 to 20 minutes.

3 / Remove with warm water and a washcloth, wiping gently to remove. (If you notice any yellow discoloration from the turmeric, don't fret! Just wash with a gentle foaming cleanser.)

4 / Finish with a moisturizer.

Tip / No time for a full-on mask? Just massage the mixture over clean, damp skin, moving up from your chin in small circles. Then rinse and moisturize.

Beauty Inside Out

Turmeric is as good for your health as it is for your skin. Rich in curcumin (an antioxidant that triggers serotonin and dopamine production), this flavorful spice is a natural mood booster. It's also antibacterial, antiseptic, and anti-inflammatory! Here's how to incorporate it into your diet.

MORNING SMOOTHIE Combine 1 cup (250 g) pineapple, 1 cup (240 mL) coconut water, a 1-inch- (2.5-cm-) long piece of fresh ginger root, and ¼ teaspoon turmeric in a blender and pulse together. Top with a squeeze of lime.

GOLDEN MILK This rich, soothing milk has been a mainstay of Ayurvedic medicine for thousands of years. To prepare the paste, mix ¼ cup (40 g) turmeric and ½ cup (120 mL) water in a small saucepan. Stir for 7 to 10 minutes over medium heat. Combine 2 teaspoons of the resulting paste with 4 cups (945 mL) coconut milk in a medium saucepan and stir over medium heat until warm. Drink 1 cup (240 mL) every night, sweetening if desired.

MATERIALS	TOOLS	RECOMMENDED FOR	STORAGE ADVICE
2 tablespoons rice flour (or ground oats if your skin is dry)	**Measuring spoons**	**All skin types**	**Use immediately**
1 teaspoon turmeric spice	**Small bowl**	FREQUENCY OF USE	
1 teaspoon honey	**Spoon**	**1 to 2 times per week**	
3 tablespoons milk or organic, full-fat, plain yogurt	**Washcloth**		
	Foaming cleanser (optional)		

Try Multimasking

Ladies with combination skin, take heart: You can use different masks at the same time to treat the needs of different areas of your face. This turmeric mask is great for dry spots (like your cheeks), but try customizing it by adding a clay mask for your T-zone and carrot mask to fight fine lines around your eyes.

Green Tea

No doubt you've heard the many benefits of drinking green tea. But let's talk about putting the wonder ingredient to work for your face! The antioxidants in green tea work to repair skin and help protect it from the damaging effects of the sun. Plus, green tea's natural tannins and anti-inflammatory powers soothe irritation and redness—and we can all drink to that!

MATCHA GREEN TEA FACIAL

1 tablespoon matcha green tea powder
1 teaspoon honey
**Pinch of cinnamon
(not for sensitive skin)**
½ tablespoon water

Mix the matcha tea powder, honey, and cinnamon in a small bowl, adding the water slowly until you reach a consistency thick enough to slather on. Spread on your face (avoiding the eye area) and neck, then relax for 20 minutes. Rinse off, tone, and then moisturize.

ANTI-AGING GREEN TEA TONER

1 green tea bag
1 cup + 2 tablespoons (270 mL) distilled water
2 tablespoons pure pomegranate juice

Steep the green tea bag in 1 cup (240 mL) hot water for 5 minutes, then discard the tea bag and let it cool to room temperature. Dilute the pomegranate juice with the remaining distilled water, then mix with ¼ cup (60 mL) of the cooled green tea. Transfer the mixture to a spray bottle, and use daily after cleansing by applying with a cotton ball or spritzing all over your face and neck.

MOISTURIZING CHIA GREEN TEA FACE MASK

2 green tea bags
2 cups (470 mL) water
2 tablespoons chia seeds
3 teaspoons honey

Brew the tea and let it cool. Add the chia seeds and allow the mixture to sit for 10 minutes until it thickens, then stir in the honey. Apply ¼ cup (60 mL) of the mixture to your face with clean hands. Let the mask sit for 10 minutes and then remove with warm water, massaging your skin as you rinse. Drink the rest of the honey-chia tea.

GREEN TEA PUFFY-EYE CUBES

1 green tea bag
1 cup (240 mL) water

With plenty of antioxidants and a dose of caffeine, green tea is a perfect eye soother. You can use old tea bags on your eyes, but I like this ice treatment even more. Brew a cup of strong green tea, pour it in an ice-cube tray, and let freeze. Apply a cube to dark circles and puffy eyes—the caffeine and ice will reduce swelling and excess fluid.

Other Uses for Green Tea

GREEN TEA COOLING SPRAY

Brew 1 cup (240 mL) green tea and stick it in the refrigerator. Peel and purée ½ cucumber, then strain and discard the solids. Add 2 tablespoons cucumber juice and 1 tablespoon fresh aloe-vera gel to a small spray bottle. Use a pipette drizzle in 1 to 2 drops peppermint essential oil. Fill the rest of the bottle with green tea and shake to combine. Store in the fridge for 7 to 10 days.

REJUVENATING GREEN TEA AND LEMON BATH SOAK

After you've filled your tub with warm water, just add 3 to 5 green tea bags and ⅓ cup (80 mL) fresh lemon juice. Enjoy your soak!

CLARIFYING GREEN TEA HAIR RINSE

Heat 2 cups (470 mL) water and pour over 3 green tea bags. Steep for 10 minutes and then remove the bags. When the tea has cooled, add 2 tablespoons apple-cider vinegar. Pour over your hair in the shower after shampooing, and let it sit at least 1 minute before rinsing.

Rich Mocha Mud Mask

Three powerful ingredients team up in this luxurious mask. Bentonite clay coaxes out nasty toxins, while coffee grounds provide a little scrub action and cocoa powder delivers anti-aging antioxidants. How sweet is that!

1 / Measure and combine the cocoa powder, bentonite clay, and coffee grounds in a non-metal bowl, and stir together with a non-metal spoon. (Metal interferes with the clay's skin-detoxing powers, and you wouldn't want that! Use wood, plastic, or ceramic tools instead.)

2 / Add just enough water to make a paste.

3 / Apply the resulting mask to your face and chest with clean hands.

4 / Relax for about 15 minutes or until you feel the clay harden and dry on your cheeks, then rinse off the mask with warm water. As you rinse, gently massage the coffee grounds into your skin for a little extra exfoliation.

MATERIALS	TOOLS	FREQUENCY OF USE
1 tablespoon unsweetened cocoa powder	Non-metal measuring spoons	Weekly
1 tablespoon bentonite clay	Small non-metal bowl	
1 teaspoon finely ground coffee	Non-metal spoon	STORAGE ADVICE
Water		Use immediately
	RECOMMENDED FOR	
	All skin types	

Acai Berry + Honey Mask

When it comes to the acai berry, you can actually believe all the hype. This tiny purple wonder is chock-full of vitamins A, C, and E, which work together to stave off free radicals and even, brighten, and tighten your face.

1 / Measure out the acai-berry powder, Manuka honey, and olive oil, and mix them with a spoon in a small bowl. (What's Manuka honey, you ask? Native to New Zealand, it's a medicinal version of the usual sweet stuff.)

2 / Apply the pretty purple mixture to clean skin and let it sit for 10 to 15 minutes.

3 / Rinse with warm water and a washcloth to remove. Finish off with a moisturizer.

Tip / The acai berry's benefits go more than skin deep. Packed with antioxidants, it aids in digestive ailments, lowers cholesterol, kick-starts weight loss, improves circulation, and more. So put some in a smoothie today!

MATERIALS	TOOLS	FREQUENCY OF USE
1 tablespoon acai-berry powder	Measuring spoons	Weekly
1 teaspoon Manuka honey	Spoon	
1 tablespoon olive oil	Small bowl	STORAGE ADVICE
	Washcloth	Use immediately
	RECOMMENDED FOR	
	Dry, aging, or normal skin	

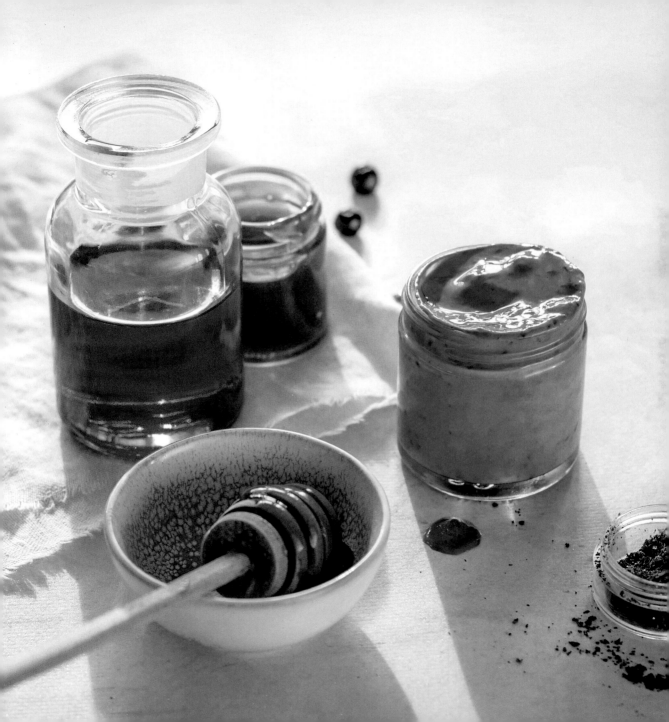

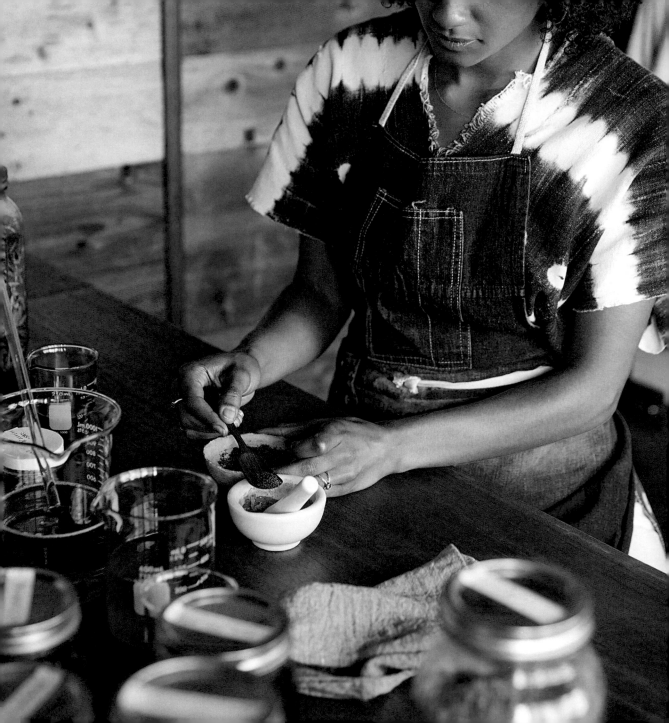

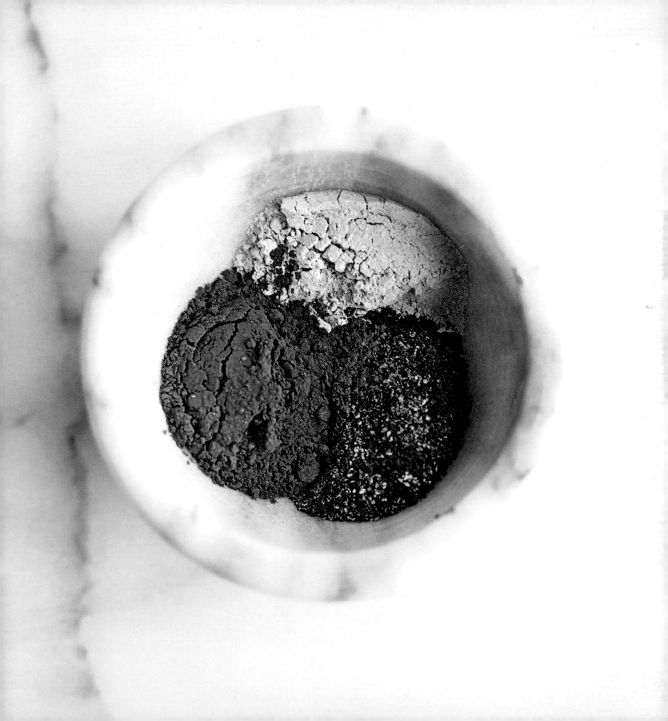

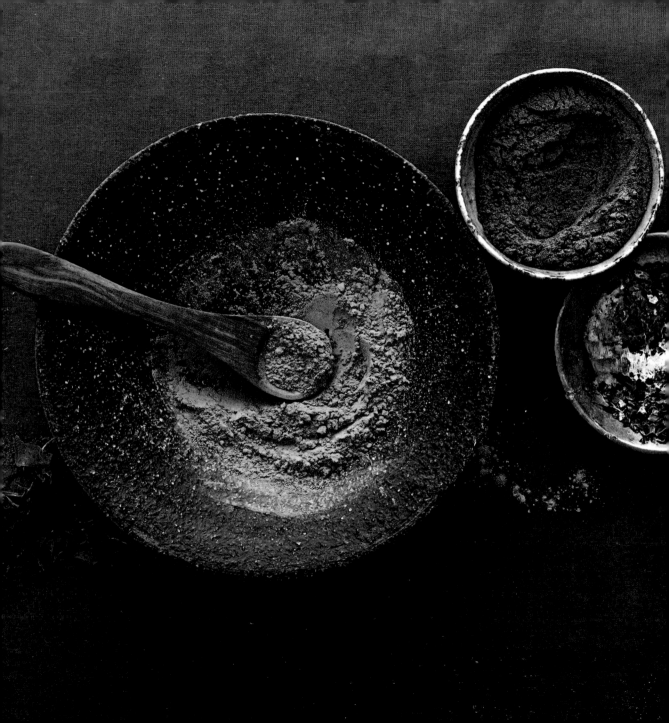

French Green Clay +Sea Kelp Mask

Clay masks are great skin detoxifiers—they work to minimize pores, control oil, and remove dead skin cells. Mineral-rich sea kelp also helps clear out blemishes, while spirulina—with four times the antioxidants found in berries!—is a formidable opponent in fighting free radicals and fine lines. Mix up the "mud" with coconut milk for a skin-softening and soothing treat.

1 / Using a plastic or ceramic measuring spoon, portion out the clay. (Again, we want to avoid metal tools, which can interfere with the clay.) Transfer to a small non-metal bowl.

2 / Measure and add the sea-kelp and spirulina powders. Stir well with a non-metal spoon to mix it all up.

3 / Transfer the mixture to a small jar. Pop on the lid and store your concoction in a cool, dry spot.

4 / When you're ready to use, pour 1 to 2 teaspoons of the powdered ingredients into a small non-metal bowl. Add the coconut milk until you get a smooth, mudlike consistency and texture.

5 / Apply the mask with clean fingers, avoiding the eye area. Leave the mask on for 15 to 20 minutes, then rinse off with warm water.

Know Your Clays

Go ahead, get some mud on your face! Clay is famous for drawing out impurities, improving circulation, and tightening up skin. A simple mix of clay and water makes a great cleanser or mask—pick one that works for you!

WHITE KAOLIN CLAY Also called cosmetic or China clay, this stuff is the mildest of all clays—wonderful for sensitive skin. It stimulates circulation and exfoliates, but it doesn't draw oils from the pores.

BENTONITE CLAY This easy-to-find clay comes from volcanic ash sediments and is supereffective at pulling out toxins. It's best for normal to oily skin.

FRENCH GREEN CLAY Also called sea clay, this highly absorbent green mud boasts essential minerals, iron oxides, and plant matter, such as kelp and seaweed. It's great for normal to oily skin—try it on trouble spots or zits.

RED CLAY Ideal for oily and acne-prone skin, red (or rhassoul) clay hails from Morocco. This mineral-rich clay is loaded with silica and magnesium—it busts up blackheads and unclogs pores.

MATERIALS

2 ounces (60 g) French green clay

1 teaspoon sea-kelp powder

1 teaspoon spirulina powder

1 to 2 tablespoons coconut milk

TOOLS

Non-metal measuring spoons

Small non-metal bowl

Non-metal spoon

3-ounce (90-mL) glass jar with plastic lid

RECOMMENDED FOR

All skin types

FREQUENCY OF USE

Up to 2 times per week

STORAGE ADVICE

Store dry ingredients for up to 1 year

Banana Face Smoothie

Move over, banana bread! Turn that browning fruit into a treat for parched skin that's full of good fats, vitamins, and potassium, plus cinnamon to open up pores for improved penetration of nutrients.

1 / Add the banana and avocado to a blender or food processor. Measure and add the cinnamon, followed by a liquid of your choosing. You can go with water, a floral hydrosol (an aromatic liquid made by distilling botanicals), a veggie juice (like carrot), or a non-dairy milk like soy milk. Avoid acidic liquids, such as fruit juices.

2 / Blend to create a smooth paste, then transfer to a small bowl.

3 / To use, apply the mask to a clean face with your fingers.

4 / Let the mask sit for 15 to 20 minutes, then rinse off with warm water.

Tip / The cinnamon in your spice rack has a secret—it's great for plumping skin, including lips! Mix a little with coconut oil and dab onto your mouth for a fuller look.

MATERIALS	TOOLS	FREQUENCY OF USE
1 medium banana	Blender or food processor	2 to 3 times per week
½ avocado	Measuring spoons	
1 teaspoon cinnamon	Small bowl	STORAGE ADVICE
2 tablespoons non-acidic liquid of your choosing	RECOMMENDED FOR	Refrigerate covered and use within 2 to 3 days
	Normal to dry skin	

Pineapple-Papaya Mask

If an esthetician suggests laser treatment for sun-damaged skin, here's a second opinion. This delightfully tropical option combines enzymes from two fruits to remove dead skin layers, reducing age spots and wrinkles.

1 / Halve the papaya, then peel, seed, and chop it into cubes, about 1 cup (140 g). Cut away one-third of the pineapple and chop into chunks—you should have 1 cup (185 g). Combine the papaya and pineapple by juicing, mashing, or pulsing them in a juicer or a blender.

2 / Filter the juice into a small bowl by pouring the mixture through a fine-mesh strainer. Discard the pulp (or enjoy it as a snack!) and add the honey, if using.

3 / First wash your chest, neck, and face. Then use cotton balls to apply the mask, avoiding the eye area.

4 / Lie down and let the scrub work its magic for 10 to 15 minutes. Be warned, it will tingle and itch a little.

5 / Rinse with warm water and moisturize. So long, unwanted discoloration and freckles!

MATERIALS	TOOLS	FREQUENCY OF USE
1 fresh papaya	Knife	1 to 2 times per week
1 fresh pineapple	Measuring cup and spoon	
1 tablespoon honey (optional)	Juicer or blender	STORAGE ADVICE
	Small bowl	Refrigerate covered and use within 7 to 10 days
	Fine-mesh strainer	
	Cotton balls	
	RECOMMENDED FOR	
	Normal or mature skin	

Use It All Up

If you've got time, slather this summery treat on the backs of your hands, which are typically the first areas of the body to show the telltale signs of aging. Still got extra? Freeze it in ice-cube trays for a rainy day when you could use a dose of island life.

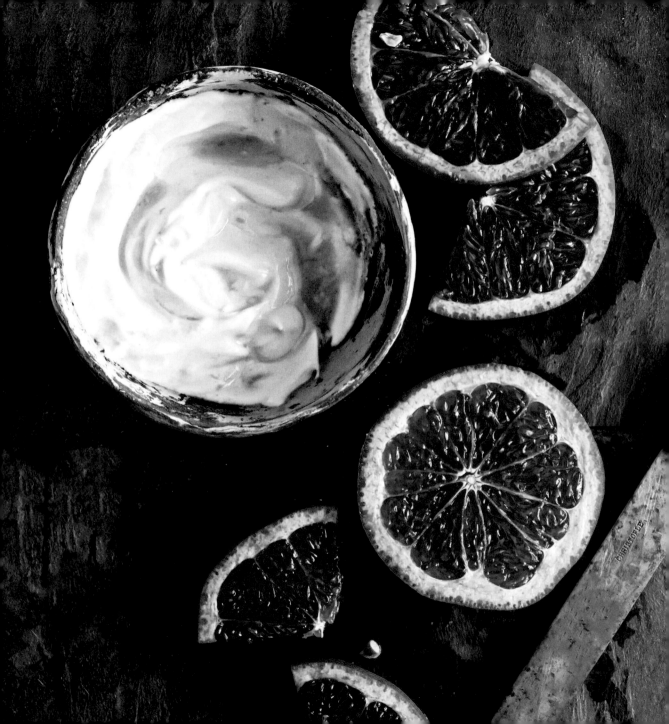

Grapefruit Detox Mask

Like lemons, grapefruits are loaded with natural acids that exfoliate dead skin, keeping your pores clean and complexion bright. Grapefruits also contain retinol antioxidants, which fight the free radicals that cause wrinkles, discoloration, and dull complexion. This recipe's healthy helping of yogurt also moisturizes and exfoliates, while its probiotics fight acne and inflammation.

1 / At the grocery store, look for the darkest red or pink grapefruit you can find. Its color indicates the presence of more lycopene, the chemical that provides most of this recipe's regenerating antioxidant power.

2 / Cut the grapefruit in half and then squeeze one of the halves into a bowl. (Better eat that remaining grapefruit—it's high in vitamin C and fiber!) Add the yogurt and use a spoon to mix.

3 / Apply a thick layer of the mixture to clean skin. This mask can get drippy, so lie down to prevent it from running into your eyes or making a mess. Leave the mask on for up to 10 minutes.

4 / Rinse with warm water, then follow with moisturizer.

Tip / Grapefruit can also act as a diuretic, so try this mask next time you're dealing with facial puffiness.

Beauty Inside Out

Chances are, you don't need me to tell you about the incredible health benefits of citrus. Grapefruit in particular is thought to help keep skin clear and trigger weight loss, as well as lower the risk of diabetes and heart disease. Get it in your diet to experience its many perks.

FLAT BELLY DETOX WATER
Cut 1 grapefruit, 1 tangerine, and 1 cucumber into thin slices. Add them to 1 gallon (3¾ L) water and mix in 10 to 20 fresh peppermint leaves. Refrigerate for 4 to 6 hours, serve over ice, and drink all day to flush the belly bloat away.

LIVER CLEANSE SMOOTHIE In addition to grapefruit, dandelion leaves and parsley are the stars in this creamy detox smoothie. They help purge the liver, while cayenne and radish spice things up. Peel ½ grapefruit and chop ½ cup (20 g) fresh parsley. Put both into a blender with 1 cup (60 g) chopped spinach, 1½ cups (360 mL) dairy-free milk, 3 dandelion leaves, 1 radish, and a dash of cayenne. Blend until smooth and then slurp down at once!

MATERIALS	TOOLS	RECOMMENDED FOR	STORAGE ADVICE
½ red or pink grapefruit	Knife	All skin types	Use immediately
½ cup (125 g) organic, full-fat, plain yogurt	Small bowl		
	Measuring cup	FREQUENCY OF USE	
	Spoon	Weekly	

Calming Aloe Vera +Lemon Face Pack

Aloe vera and lemon juice are both rich in vitamins A, C, and E—together, they make one fantastic face pack. In this mask, the succulent's healing superpowers clear skin while reducing inflammation and pain, while the lemon juice's mighty citric acid acts as a natural exfoliant that gently peels away the top layers of dead skin—taking pigmentation and acne scars along with them. Good riddance!

1 / Cut two aloe-vera leaves from the base of your plant. Slice off the pointy edges, then chop the leaf into 2- to 3-inch (5–7.5-cm) sections. (This process makes accessing the gel much easier than slicing an entire leaf.) Once you've opened up the leaf, use a knife to extract the gel. It's okay if you get some pulp too.

2 / Cut the lemon in half and squeeze the juice out of one half, then mix the liquid with the gel (plus any attached pulp) and honey in a blender. Blend for 1 minute. Transfer to a small bowl.

3 / Apply the mixture directly to your face and neck, and leave on for between 10 and 15 minutes. Or soak a thin cloth in the mix, then drape it over your face and neck for 20 minutes.

4 / Remove the mask with warm water and follow with moisturizer.

All About That Aloe

If you keep one plant on your kitchen windowsill, make it aloe. This marvelous succulent crops up in natural beauty, first aid, and meal recipes all the time. Here are some simple ones to try out!

SUNBURN SOOTHER Fresh aloe vera straight from the plant does wonders for sunburns. Just split a leaf in half, squeeze out the juice, and add a little vitamin E. Then apply directly to the burn. Ah!

HYDRATING ALOE WATER Cut 2 leaves in half lengthwise, then scoop out the translucent gel and add it to a blender. Add 1 cup (240 mL) coconut water and ½ cucumber, roughly chopped. Pulse and strain to remove the cuke chunks, then consume right away for a vitamin- and antioxidant-rich drink.

DEWY DIY SERUM Combine fresh-off-the-plant aloe-vera gel with a carrier oil that works for your skin type (I use jojoba) and a few drops of essential oil. The result? A healing, hydrating, and lightweight homemade face serum that's perfect for daytime.

MATERIALS

2 aloe-vera leaves

1 lemon

1 tablespoon honey

TOOLS

Knife

Measuring spoons

Blender

Small bowl

Thin cloth (optional)

RECOMMENDED FOR

All skin types

FREQUENCY OF USE

1 to 2 times per week

STORAGE ADVICE

Refrigerate covered and use within 7 to 10 days

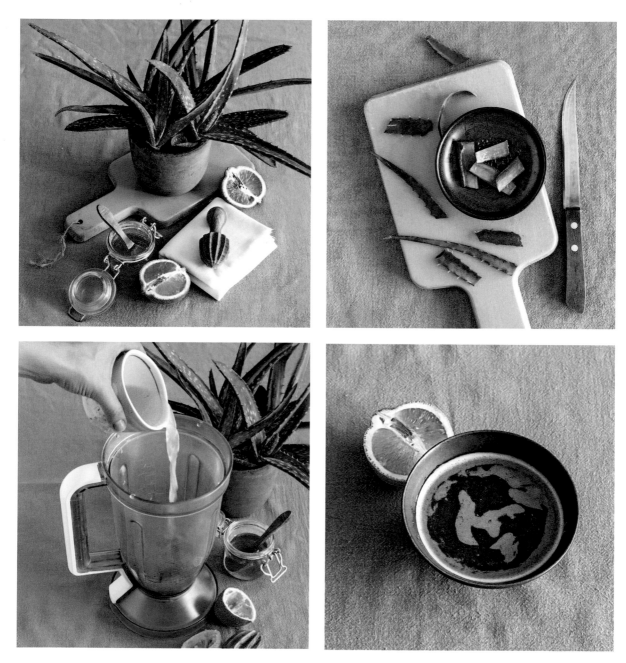

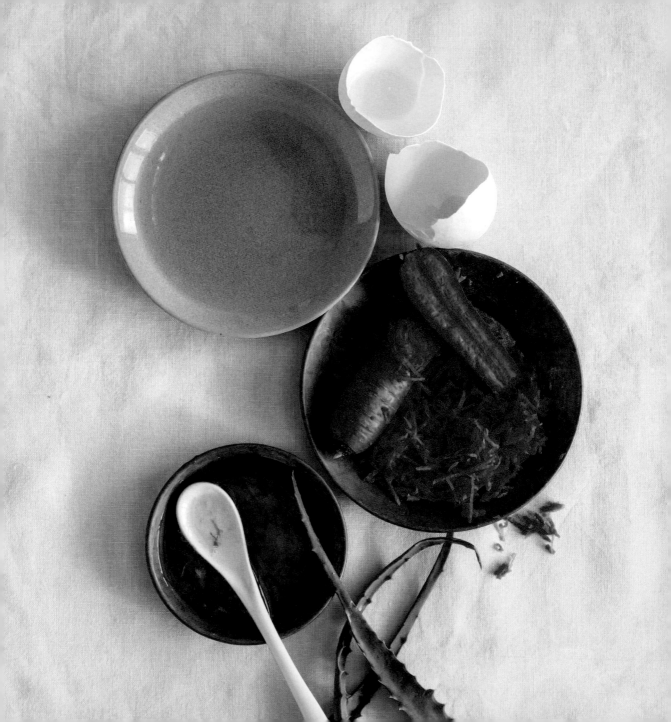

Carrot+Egg Eye Mask

The vitamins and proteins in egg whites firm up the skin, which is especially effective on pesky crow's feet. Plus, carrots' beta-carotene is a natural way to treat yourself to retinol, one of the best wrinkle-fighting ingredients.

1 / Grate the carrot so it's finely shredded. (Steer clear of baby carrots—they lose most natural nutrients when processed.) Measure out 1 tablespoon shredded carrot and reserve the rest—hello, lunchtime salad!

2 / Separate the egg white from the yolk. Combine the egg white, shredded carrot, and aloe-vera gel in a small bowl; beat with a fork for 1 minute so it's nice and frothy.

3 / With your hands or a makeup brush, apply the mask around and under the eyes. Avoid the eyelids—trust me.

4 / Let the mask dry for 15 to 30 minutes. You will definitely feel it hardening—it's okay to remove if it gets too tight. To do so, lay a wet towel over your eyes to remoisten, then wipe off the mask and moisturize.

MATERIALS	TOOLS	RECOMMENDED FOR
1 carrot	Grater	All skin types
1 egg	Measuring spoons	
1 teaspoon fresh aloe-vera gel	Small bowl	**FREQUENCY OF USE**
	Fork	Weekly
	Makeup brush (optional)	**STORAGE ADVICE**
	Towel	Use immediately

Longer-Lash Serum

Make your lashes shinier and fuller with this supereasy, two-ingredient serum. The fatty acids and vitamin E in castor oil strengthen the lash root and stimulate growth, while the aloe-vera gel conditions to prevent breakage.

1 / Measure and combine the castor oil and aloe-vera gel in a small container with a lid.

2 / Shake before each use to make sure the ingredients are well combined.

3 / Apply to your lashes with a Q-tip or a clean mascara wand every night before you go to bed. Resist the urge to rinse it off—instead, let it seep in overnight and work its magic. Use this serum for 2 weeks, and you'll start to see a reduction in lash breakage.

Tip / For even stronger lashes, make sure to get some vitamin E in your diet (think nuts and seeds!). And for extra lash nourishment, drizzle a few drops of olive oil or vitamin E oil into the lash serum.

MATERIALS	TOOLS	FREQUENCY OF USE
2 tablespoons castor oil	Measuring spoon	Daily
2 tablespoons fresh aloe-vera gel	2-ounce (60-mL) lidded jar	**STORAGE ADVICE**
	Q-tip or clean mascara wand	Use within 3 months
	RECOMMENDED FOR	
	All skin types	

Caffeine-Fix Eye Cream

When no amount of concealer can cover up a late night, try a simple—but effective—caffeine eye cream to rescue those tired peepers. A potent antioxidant that helps repair aging skin, caffeine also reduces swelling while increasing blood flow. Pair it up with cooling witch hazel, a natural astringent that also alleviates puffiness.

1 / Measure and pour the fresh coffee grounds into your glass jar. Add the sweet almond oil too.

2 / Replace the lid on the jar and shake thoroughly to disperse the oil throughout the grounds.

3 / Let the jar sit in a sunny spot for 2 to 5 days, shaking it once a day. (Infusing oil with this solar method can take time. If you want to complete this project faster, infuse the grounds with the heat method instead—flip to page 38 for a description.)

4 / Using a fine-mesh strainer, filter the coffee-oil mixture into a heat-safe glass bowl. Discard the grounds.

5 / Add the beeswax to the coffee-oil solution. Place the bowl in a small saucepan of water and heat it until the wax is fully melted.

6 / Remove the mixture from heat and allow it to cool to a lukewarm temperature.

7 / Empty the water from the pan and add the witch hazel. Heat it until it's lukewarm, then pour it into a medium bowl. Beat with a hand mixer on medium while adding the coffee-oil mixture in a slow and steady stream.

8 / Continue beating the witch hazel and the coffee-oil mixture together until a creamy emulsion forms, then transfer to the larger lidded jar.

9 / Apply around and underneath the eye area for a quick pick-me-up. Keep in the fridge between uses—this cream is even more effective when it's cold.

Tip / If you don't end up with ½ cup of the coffee-oil mixture after straining, just top it off with a little almond oil.

MATERIALS

¼ cup (50 g) fresh coffee grounds

½ cup (120 mL) sweet almond oil

½ ounce (15 g) beeswax

6 tablespoons witch hazel

TOOLS

Measuring cup

6-ounce (180-mL) lidded glass jar

Fine-mesh strainer

Small heat-safe glass bowl

Small saucepan

Medium bowl

Hand mixer

8-ounce (240-mL) lidded glass jar

RECOMMENDED FOR

All skin types

FREQUENCY OF USE

Daily

STORAGE ADVICE

Refrigerate and use within 3 months

MORE FIXES FOR PUFFY EYES

ELEVATE YOUR HEAD Sleep with your head propped up on a pillow to prevent excess fluid buildup.

GO COLD Soak a washcloth in cold water, wring it out, and lay it over your eyes to restrict blood flow and nix swelling. Or refrigerate two spoons and hold them over your eyes in the a.m.

REDUCE SALT Extra salt leads to water retention, which can cause puffiness.

TRY TATERS We've all put cucumber slices on our eyes. The same trick works with raw potatoes!

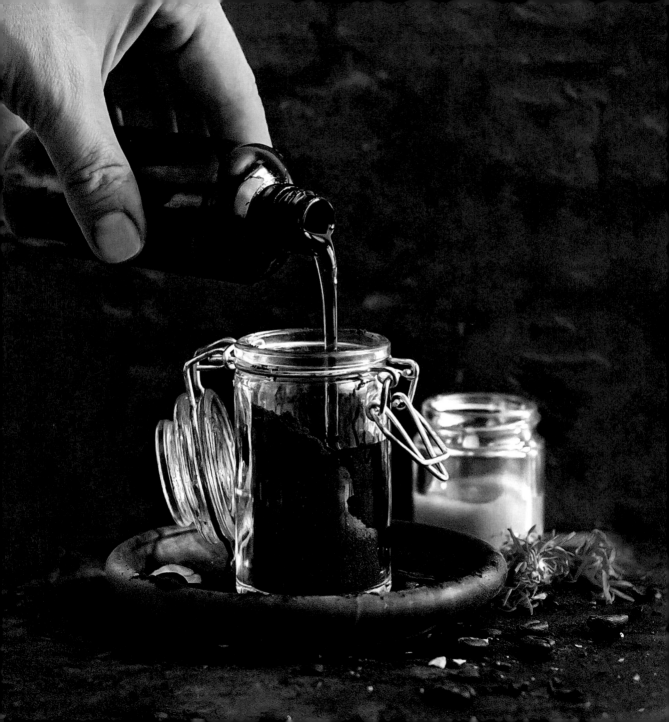

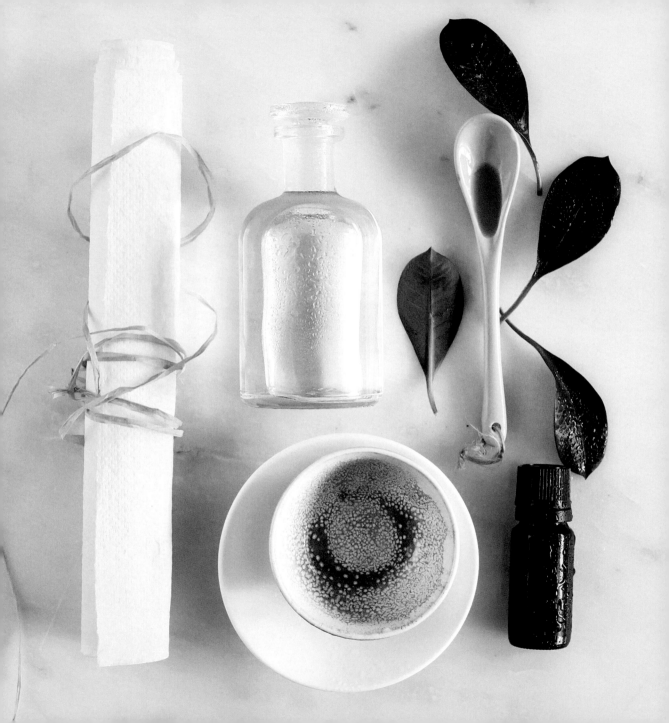

Eye-Makeup Remover Wipes

Sleeping in mascara, eyeliner, and eyeshadow clogs up your pores, puts you at risk for eye infections, and causes premature aging. So cut it out! Remove all your eye makeup with these easy-to-make and even easier-to-use wipes.

1 / Measure and mix the witch hazel, jojoba oil, and water in a small bowl. Add the tea-tree oil with a pipette.

2 / Use a serrated knife to cut the roll of paper towels in half width-wise. Remove the tube from one half.

3 / Put the half without the tube in an airtight container, then pour the solution over the roll. (Need more to cover the wipes? Increase the witch hazel, jojoba oil, and water in a 1:1:1 ratio, then add 1 to 2 drops tea-tree oil.)

4 / Replace the lid and turn the container upside down to make sure the other side of the roll gets soaked too.

5 / Store with the lid on to keep the wipes from drying. To use, pull wipes from the roll's center and clean off your eye makeup before bed. See—lazy can look good!

MATERIALS	TOOLS	FREQUENCY OF USE
2 tablespoons witch hazel	Measuring spoon	Daily
2 tablespoons jojoba oil	Small bowl	
2 tablespoons distilled water	Pipette	STORAGE ADVICE
1 to 2 drops tea-tree oil	Serrated knife	Use within 3 months
Roll of paper towels	1-quart (1-L) lidded plastic container	

RECOMMENDED FOR

All skin types

Silky Avocado Eye Cream

Glance at the label on a jar of fancy eye cream—it likely contains avocado oil, which is rich in wrinkle-fighting vitamin E. Mix it with shea butter for a creamy texture that glides on without feeling greasy.

1 / Measure the shea butter into a small glass jar.

2 / Bring 2 inches (5 cm) of water to boil in a small saucepan and lower the heat, then place the glass jar in the saucepan. Wait for the shea butter to melt, stirring occasionally with a spoon.

3 / Once the shea butter has melted, remove the jar from the water bath. Let it cool for 2 to 3 minutes.

4 / Measure and add the avocado and vitamin E oils. Stir to combine, then continue stirring while the mixture cools to create a smooth, creamy texture.

5 / Replace the lid and store the cream in a cool, dry spot. To use, apply a little to the outer corners of your eyes by gently tapping, not tugging, the skin.

MATERIALS	TOOLS	FREQUENCY OF USE
1 tablespoon shea butter	Measuring spoons	Daily
1 tablespoon avocado oil	1-ounce (30-mL) lidded glass jar	
1 teaspoon vitamin E oil	Small saucepan	STORAGE ADVICE
	Spoon	Use within 6 months

RECOMMENDED FOR

All skin types

Berries

Not only are berries a tasty treat, they're also loaded with vitamins, minerals, and antioxidants that nourish your skin. Plus, they have tons of vitamin C, which gives your face a major boost by destroying free radicals and assisting in collagen production. These little powerhouses also pack a punch in alpha hydroxy acids, which exfoliate dead epidermal cells and make berries perfect for dull or acne-prone skin. So save a few from the pie heap for these simple beauty recipes!

BERRY-YOGURT AGE-FIGHTING MASK

2 tablespoons organic, full-fat, plain yogurt
2 tablespoons honey
¼ cup (25 g) mixed berries

In a blender, combine the yogurt, honey, and mixed berries—try blackberries, strawberries, blueberries, whatever the farmers' market bin has to offer. Pulse until they're all smooth and combined. Apply to clean skin with your hands; leave on for 10 to 20 minutes before rinsing off.

GENTLE BLUEBERRY-OATMEAL CLEANSER

2 tablespoons oatmeal
2 tablespoons blueberries
Water (optional)

Toss the oatmeal and antioxidant-rich blueberries in a blender, and pulse until combined and coarsely ground. Make a paste, adding water if needed, and gently apply to your face by moving your fingers in small circles. Rinse with warm water.

ZIT-ZAPPING STRAWBERRY FACE PEEL

3 to 5 non-coated aspirin
1 tablespoon lemon juice
1 strawberry

To benefit from aspirin's acne-fighting salicylic acid, crush the pills into a fine powder, then add the fresh lemon juice. Let the pills dissolve. Mash the strawberry and stir it into the mixture. Dip a cotton ball into the liquid and apply to your face, avoiding the eyes. Leave the peel on for 10 to 15 minutes, then rinse with warm water.

WHITENING STRAWBERRY TEETH SCRUB

1 strawberry
1 teaspoon baking soda

Mash the strawberry and combine it with the baking soda in a small bowl. Dip a toothbrush or your finger into the mixture and brush your teeth for 1 to 2 minutes. Rinse thoroughly and finish with regular flossing and brushing. Repeat twice a month for a whiter smile.

Other Uses for Berries

BRIGHTENING ALMOND-STRAWBERRY BODY SCRUB

Combine 3 to 4 mashed strawberries in a small bowl, then top it off with ¾ cup (150 g) brown sugar and ¼ cup (60 mL) sweet almond oil. Stir and apply the mixture in circular motions all over your body before showering.

SO-VERY-BERRY HAIR MASK

Measure 2 tablespoons each raspberries, blueberries, and blackberries, then toss them in a blender and pulse with water to make a paste. Apply the resulting paste directly to wet hair and let it sit for between 10 and 15 minutes. The antioxidants will fight damaging environmental effects on hair, leaving it shiny and voluminous.

DELICIOUS BLUEBERRY-POMEGRANATE INFUSION

For a great way to hydrate from the inside out, infuse ¼ cup (30 g) blueberries in 20 ounces (590 mL) water for an hour, then add ½ teaspoon sea salt and 2 tablespoons pomegranate juice. Bottoms up!

Lavender-Pomegranate Lip Balm

Looking to make your own beauty products? DIY lip balm is the perfect starter project. Here, pomegranate and coconut oil deliver intensive healing, while shea butter and beeswax protect and seal in moisture.

1 / Measure the shea butter, coconut oil, and beeswax. Drop them into a small heat-safe glass bowl.

2 / Bring 2 inches (5 cm) of water to a boil in a small saucepan. Reduce the heat to low and put the bowl into the saucepan to make a water bath.

3 / Warm until the ingredients have melted together.

4 / Remove the bowl from the heat. Let the mixture cool slightly, then add the pomegranate oil and use a pipette to drizzle in the lavender essential oil. Stir with a spoon.

5 / Pour the mixture quickly into the lip balm tin. Let it rest on your countertop until it's completely cooled and hardened, then pack it everywhere you go.

MATERIALS	TOOLS	RECOMMENDED FOR
1 tablespoon shea butter	Measuring spoon	All skin types
1 tablespoon coconut oil	Small heat-safe glass bowl	**FREQUENCY OF USE**
1 tablespoon beeswax	Small saucepan	As needed
1 tablespoon pomegranate oil	Pipette	**STORAGE ADVICE**
14 drops lavender essential oil	Spoon	Use within 6 months
	2-ounce (60-mL) lip balm tin	

Scrumptious Coconut-Lime Lip Scrub

Raid the pantry to make this tasty tropical lip scrub. In under 5 minutes, you'll be gently exfoliating your lips with sugar and lime while smoothing and hydrating with coconut oil. Result? Soft, kissable lips all day!

1 / Measure the sugar and coconut oil, then combine them in a small bowl. Stir with a spoon until you have a smooth paste.

2 / Cut the lime in half and juice one half, then fold the fresh lime juice (or essential oil) into the paste.

3 / To use, apply the paste to your lips with clean fingertips. Massage gently to slough off dry, flaky skin. Rinse with warm water, then smooth that kisser with a lip balm. (Got extra scrub? Store in a lidded container.)

Tip / If your lips are sore or cracked, skip the lime and go with honey instead. This natural healer will help repair skin and lock in moisture.

MATERIALS	TOOLS	FREQUENCY OF USE
1 tablespoon sugar	Measuring spoon	Up to 2 times per week
1 tablespoon coconut oil	Small bowl	**STORAGE ADVICE**
1 lime (or 1 drop lime essential oil)	Spoon	Refrigerate and use within 1 week
Honey (optional)	Knife	
	1-ounce (30-mL) lidded container	

RECOMMENDED FOR

All skin types

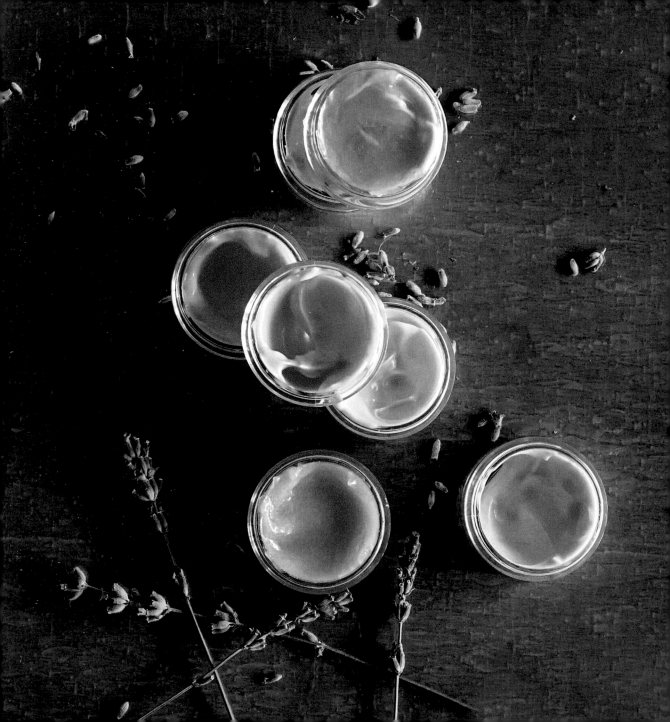

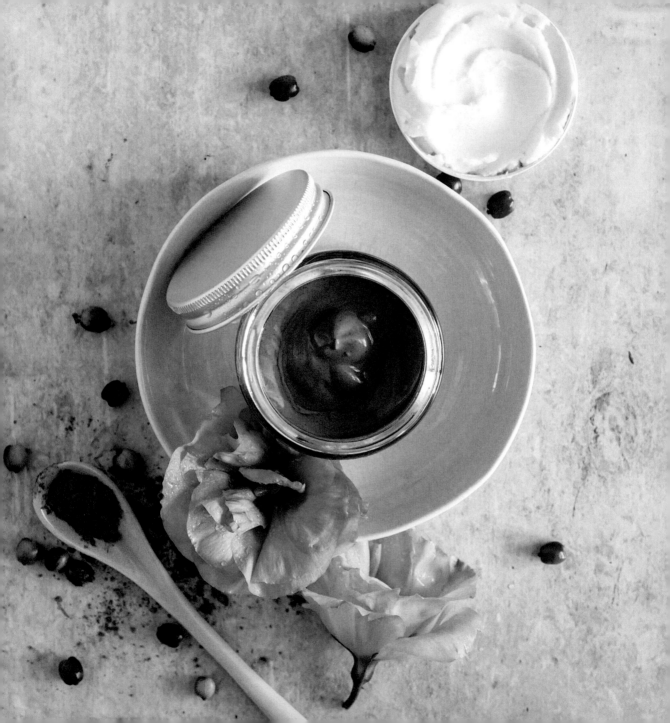

Cranberry Lip Gloss + Cheek Stain

Making your own beauty products can be addictive, especially when they turn out as pretty as this double-duty lip gloss and cheek stain. It looks almost good enough to eat, and guess what? It is! How many commercial blushes or lip glosses can say that? The gloss melts easily into the skin on contact, leaving a hint of shine and color.

1 / Measure out the coconut oil and drop it into a small heat-safe glass bowl. Set it inside a small saucepan.

2 / Pour 2 inches (5 cm) of water into the saucepan and heat it on low.

3 / Once the coconut oil has melted, measure and add the cranberry and beetroot powders. Let the mixture stand for 1 hour to infuse the oil, monitoring the saucepan and adding more water if needed. Remove from heat and let the mixture cool slightly.

4 / Strain the warm oil through the cheesecloth into a small bowl. Press gently on the solids to extract as much of the oil as possible, then discard the leftover liquid.

5 / Stir in the shea butter. It should melt easily if the oil is still warm.

(If not, gently warm the oils over low heat until melted, then remove the oil-butter mixture from heat.)

6 / Let the mixture cool, stirring to keep the color particles suspended.

7 / When it's solidified, gently beat it with a spoon until light and creamy.

8 / Transfer to a small jar with a tight-fitting lid and use whenever you could stand a touch of color.

Tip / This gloss melts easily, so don't keep it in your pocket! If you live in a warm climate, you can add a small amount of beeswax to firm up your gloss and add more texture. Melt ½ teaspoon beeswax pellets into the coconut oil after straining to give it a more balm-like consistency, then finish cooling and beating the cream.

MATERIALS

2 tablespoons coconut oil

1 tablespoon freeze-dried cranberry powder

½ teaspoon beetroot powder

1 to 2 teaspoons shea butter

½ teaspoon beeswax pellets (optional)

TOOLS

Measuring spoons

Small heat-safe glass bowl

Small saucepan

Cheesecloth

Small bowl

Spoon

1-ounce (30-mL) lidded glass jar

RECOMMENDED FOR

All skin types

FREQUENCY OF USE

As needed

STORAGE ADVICE

Store in lidded container and use within 6 months

MORE COLOR IDEAS FOR LIP/CHEEK STAINS

CHERRIES Pit 3 cherries and mash them in a small bowl. Mix their juices in with 1 teaspoon glycerin, and apply to your lips and cheeks. Works with berries and pomegranates too!

FAVORITE LIPSTICKS You can add color to any lip gloss by mixing in a small piece of lipstick (preferably an all-natural one). Powder blush or eye shadow also works great.

RED BEETS Roasting brings out the gorgeous color of these root veggies. Cook for 30 to 50 minutes at 350°F (175°C) until soft. Let cool completely and then rub a small piece on your lips.

All-Natural Customizable Beetroot Blush

With this supereasy powder blush, there's no one "right" way—which means there's no wrong way, either! Working with just two or three ingredients, you can experiment to find the shade that works best for you.

1 / Add the arrowroot flour or cornstarch to a bowl. (Cornstarch is more common, but may contain GMOs.)

2 / Start with 1 tablespoon beetroot powder, then add more until you like the color. Equal parts beetroot and arrowroot will give a lighter blush, while a 2:1 beetroot-arrowroot ratio will give you a darker, more true pink. Experiment with mixing equal parts turmeric, beetroot, and arrowroot for a peach-colored blush, or add cocoa powder to darken the hue.

3 / Mix the powders with a spoon to break up clumps, then transfer to a lidded jar and store in a dry place.

4 / To use, just dip a brush into the powder, tap off the excess, and apply to the apples of your cheeks.

MATERIALS	TOOLS	FREQUENCY OF USE
1 tablespoon arrowroot flour or cornstarch	Measuring spoons	Daily
Beetroot powder	Small bowl	
Turmeric (optional)	Spoon	STORAGE ADVICE
Unsweetened cocoa powder (optional)	3-ounce (80-mL) lidded jar	Use within 6 months
	Blush brush	
	RECOMMENDED FOR	
	All skin types	

Sun-Kissed Foundation Powder

Forget roasting in the sun for hours, trying to achieve that coveted summertime glow at a risk to your health. Instead, use this simple formula to put a little color in your cheeks, or even to contour and sculpt your face.

1 / Measure and mix the cocoa powder with the arrowroot flour or cornstarch in a small bowl. Test the color on your skin over your usual foundation or powder.

2 / Sprinkle in more cocoa powder or cornstarch to darken or lighten. For a little glimmer, try adding a pinch of cinnamon, nutmeg, turmeric, or beetroot powder.

3 / When you're happy with the color, blend with a spoon and transfer to a jar. Store in a dry place.

4 / Dip a brush into the powder, tapping off any excess before applying to your cheeks. To contour, apply the powder in a wedge shape under the cheekbones. The long edge of the triangle should start at the ear and taper out under the apple or middle of the cheek.

MATERIALS	TOOLS	FREQUENCY OF USE
1 tablespoon cocoa powder	Measuring spoons	Daily
1 teaspoon arrowroot flour or cornstarch	Small bowl	
Cinnamon (optional)	Spoon	STORAGE ADVICE
Nutmeg (optional)	3-ounce (80-mL) lidded jar	Use within 6 months
Turmeric (optional)	Powder brush	
Beetroot powder (optional)	RECOMMENDED FOR	
	All skin types	

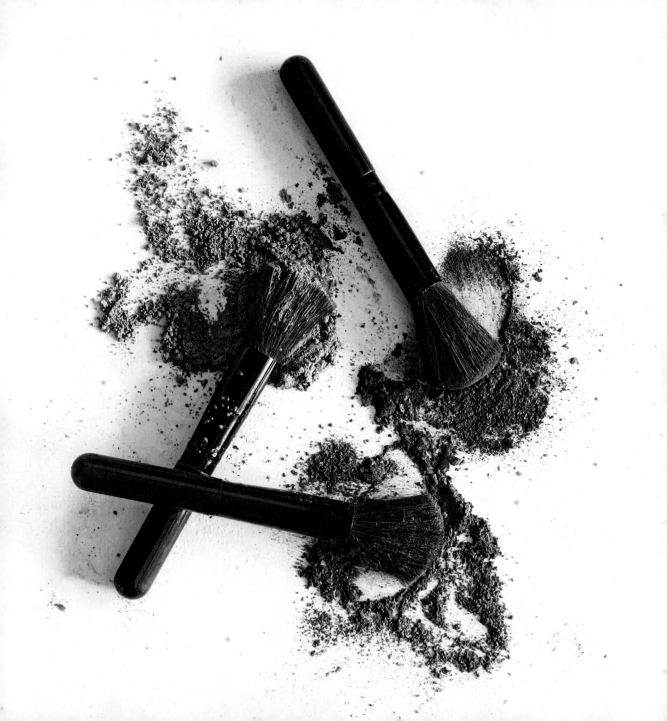

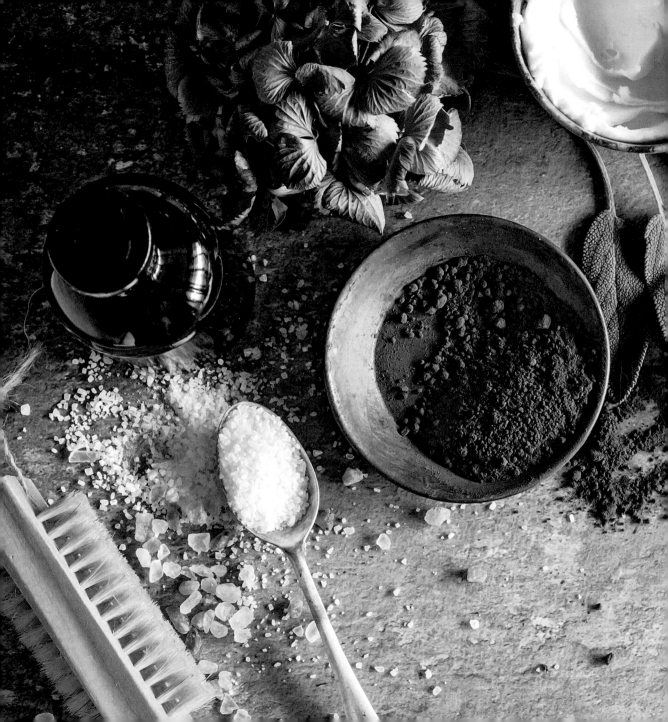

BODY

Your body works hard—better treat it right! Try this indulgent collection of soaps, perfumes, bath mixes, and more when you need some proper pampering.

BODYCARE BASICS

You likely learned in science class that your skin is your largest organ. But did you know that keeping it in good shape is a total team effort? Your organs are constantly cleansing themselves of unhealthy things—pollution, less-than-wise food choices, even stress. Reduce the burden on your body and make your skin shine more with these simple actions that detox day to day.

MORNING

1 / Rehydrate Start your day with a big mug of warm water and the juice of ½ lemon. The body loses a lot of moisture overnight, which makes water a much better choice than coffee to rehydrate your system and kick-start your bowels in the a.m. Wait on coffee until after you've eaten—caffeine causes your blood sugar to rise due to a spike in adrenaline. Food will buffer this negative effect.

2 / Dry-brush Your Skin Spend 3 to 5 minutes dry-brushing your skin with a long-handled, natural-bristle brush before your daily shower. This removes the dead layers so the body can excrete toxins more efficiently. This practice also targets the lymphatic system (think of it as your body's drainage system), which is directly beneath the skin. Use gentle pressure and brush up the body toward the lymph nodes in the armpits, groin, and neck.

3 / Power Up Breakfast Eat within the first 90 minutes of waking up to activate your metabolism and stabilize your blood sugar. Make sure your breakfast includes a serving of protein and healthy fat (like overnight oats, chia pudding, or eggs) to keep you energized. And get into a daily smoothie habit—it's an easy way to start your day right with green veggies.

EVENING

4 / Sip on Tea A warm cup of chamomile or turmeric tea signals to both your brain and body that it's time to wind down for the night. Tea's comforting effects can also help prevent you from reaching for a late-night snack. Just stick with the decaffeinated stuff.

5 / Bathe in Epsom Salts Often seen as an indulgence, a warm bath does more than comfort. Adding Epsom salt to a nightly bath removes toxins, soothes sore muscles, halts colds, and opens congested sinuses. Experiment with adding essential oils to discover what your body likes best.

6 / Stretch It Out My pre-bedtime form of meditation is to do some simple yoga, like forward bends or child's pose (a kneeling position in which you rest your bottom on your heels while touching your forehead to the floor with your arms outstretched). Or you can try putting your legs up against a wall or lying on your back in dead man's pose. It helps to shake off tension from the day and let your mind go blank for a moment—it feels so good you could fall asleep right there!

7 / Sleep Like You Mean It A good night's rest can do wonders for your skin's health. When you sleep, your body is better able to fight environmental damage, increasing its antioxidant nutrients and regenerating cells. My goal is eight hours of rest every night (hey, a girl needs her beauty sleep!). To make drifting off easy, keep a regular bedtime, turn out all the lights, and lower the room temperature when it's time to hit the hay.

ESSENTIAL OILS

They're called essential for a reason—these aromatic distillations of your favorite plants can help you sleep, ease stress, or calm a headache. To profit from their specific superpowers, select one for the change that you crave.

BALANCE

Creates a feeling of stability and improves your ability to handle stress.

Rose   Clary Sage   Geranium

INVIGORATE

Elevates energy and creates a positive outlook.

Basil   Grapefruit   Eucalyptus

FOCUS

Improves concentration and memory.

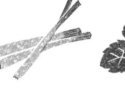

Lemongrass   Peppermint   Rosemary

DE-STRESS

Relieves tension, anxiety, and headaches.

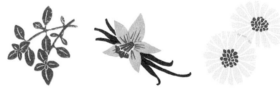

Sweet Marjoram   Vanilla   Chamomile

SERENE

Use to create peace, calm, and tranquility.

Ylang Ylang   Frankincense   Lavender

CHEER

Boosts spirits and improves mood.

Bergamot   Sandalwood   Orange

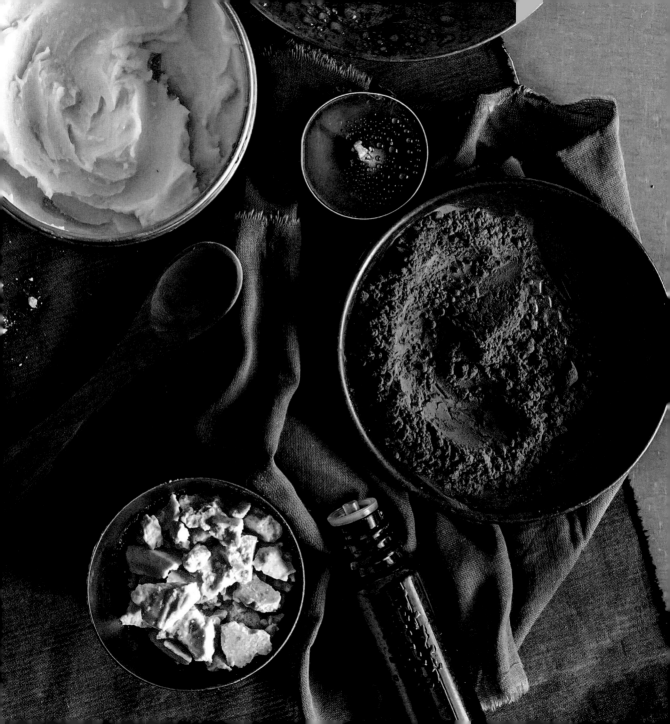

Lavish Cocoa Body Butter

This decadent cream's scent is a chocolate lover's dream, and the combination of cocoa butter and coconut oil will leave your skin nourished and silky soft. Bonus: The cocoa powder provides a hint of bronzing color.

1 / Measure the cocoa butter and coconut oil, then mix them with a spoon in a small heat-safe glass bowl.

2 / Bring 2 inches (5 cm) of water to a boil in a small saucepan, then reduce the heat to low. Place the glass bowl in the saucepan and melt the ingredients.

3 / Remove from heat and let cool for a few minutes. Stir in the cocoa powder. Add the peppermint oil with a pipette.

4 / Refrigerate for 30 minutes, until the mixture has started to set but is not yet fully hard.

5 / Blend the butter with a hand mixer on medium until fluffy, 3 to 5 minutes. Scrape down the sides as you go.

6 / Store in a lidded container in a cool, dry spot. Spread on your skin when you crave a bit of moisture.

MATERIALS	TOOLS	RECOMMENDED FOR
½ cup (110 g) cocoa butter	**Measuring cups and spoons**	**All skin types**
½ cup (100 g) coconut oil	**Spoon**	
2 tablespoons unsweetened cocoa powder	**Small heat-safe glass bowl**	**FREQUENCY OF USE**
	Small saucepan	**Daily**
5 drops peppermint essential oil	**Pipette**	
	Hand mixer	**STORAGE ADVICE**
	Rubber spatula	**Use within 6 months**
	8-ounce (240-mL) lidded container	

Stress-Melting Body Butter

Stress saps magnesium from your cells, causing anxiety, fatigue, headaches, and insomnia. You can up your daily intake with magnesium oil—and add orange, bergamot, and frankincense for a mood-boosting scent.

1 / Measure and transfer the shea butter, coconut oil, and cocoa butter to a heat-safe glass bowl. Stir to mix.

2 / Pour 2 inches (5 cm) of water into a saucepan. Bring the water to a boil, then reduce the heat to low. Put the glass bowl inside the saucepan.

3 / When the ingredients have melted, remove the bowl from the heat. Let it cool for a few minutes, then stir in the magnesium oil. Add the essential oils with a pipette.

4 / Refrigerate the bowl for 30 minutes, then remove it and whip the cream with a hand mixer on medium for 3 to 5 minutes. Scrape down the sides with a spatula.

5 / Transfer to a lidded container and keep it cool and dry. Use every night before bed for a soothing treat.

MATERIALS	TOOLS	RECOMMENDED FOR
¼ cup (50 g) shea butter	**Measuring cups**	**All skin types**
¼ cup (50 g) coconut oil	**Small heat-safe glass bowl**	
¼ cup (50 g) cocoa butter	**Spoon**	**FREQUENCY OF USE**
¼ cup (60 mL) magnesium oil	**Small saucepan**	**Daily**
10 drops orange essential oil	**Pipette**	
	Hand mixer	**STORAGE ADVICE**
10 drops bergamot essential oil	**Rubber spatula**	**Use within 6 months**
10 drops frankincense essential oil	**8-ounce (240-mL) lidded container**	

Cozy Vanilla-Chai Body Oil

Almond oil is a joy from head to toe. Rich in vitamins A, B, and E, this light oil moisturizes dehydrated, frazzled hair and soothes painful chapped lips and dry heels. Add in some black tea (which comes packed with vitamins E and C), and sprinkle the mix with cloves, cardamom, allspice, and cinnamon to create a DIY chai body oil. Oh, and vanilla—just because it smells so darn good!

1 / Measure and pour the almond oil into a heat-safe glass bowl. (If you have a nut allergy, substitute another light oil, like sunflower or grape-seed.)

2 / Bring 2 inches (5 cm) of water to a boil in a small saucepan and reduce the heat to low. Then place the glass bowl inside the saucepan and gently heat the oil.

3 / Time to add the loose tea. Black tea contains potent antioxidants, plus a dose of caffeine that helps tone skin and improve the appearance of cellulite. (Don't have black tea? A chai tea blend is a perfect substitute—you won't need all the spices either!)

4 / Measure and add the cardamom pods, whole cloves, allspice berries, and cinnamon sticks to the almond oil. Then cut open the vanilla bean and scrape the contents into the mixture.

Using vanilla beans will give you a stronger flavor and scent—along with extra antioxidants to repair skin.

5 / Continue to warm on low for 1 hour to infuse all the yummy ingredients, stirring occasionally with a spoon.

6 / Remove the bowl from heat and let it cool, then filter out the tea and spices with a fine-mesh strainer.

7 / Transfer to a pretty glass bottle with a funnel. Store in a cool, dry spot.

8 / Layer on this comforting, aromatic oil as a skin moisturizer, a massage oil, or even a makeup remover.

Tip / For a nicer presentation, try adding in some bonus whole cloves, cardamom pods, allspice berries, or cinnamon sticks to your glass bottle—it'll make a perfect autumnal treat for a friend or family member.

MATERIALS

1 cup (240 mL) sweet almond oil

¼ cup (8 g) loose black tea

1 tablespoon whole cardamom pods

1 teaspoon whole cloves

1 teaspoon allspice berries

2 cinnamon sticks

1 vanilla bean

TOOLS

Measuring cups and spoons

Small heat-safe glass bowl

Small saucepan

Knife

Spoon

Fine-mesh strainer

8-ounce (240-mL) glass bottle

Funnel

RECOMMENDED FOR

All skin types

FREQUENCY OF USE

As needed

STORAGE ADVICE

Use within 6 months

TARGETED SUBSTITUTIONS

CELLULITE
Instead of the tea and spices, gather 1 bunch fresh birch leaves and cut the peel off 2 grapefruits, then drop them into the almond oil to infuse.

SORE MUSCLES
Try 2 tablespoons sliced fresh ginger and 1 teaspoon cayenne powder.

ENERGIZING
Go with 1 bunch fresh basil leaves and the peel of 2 medium lemons.

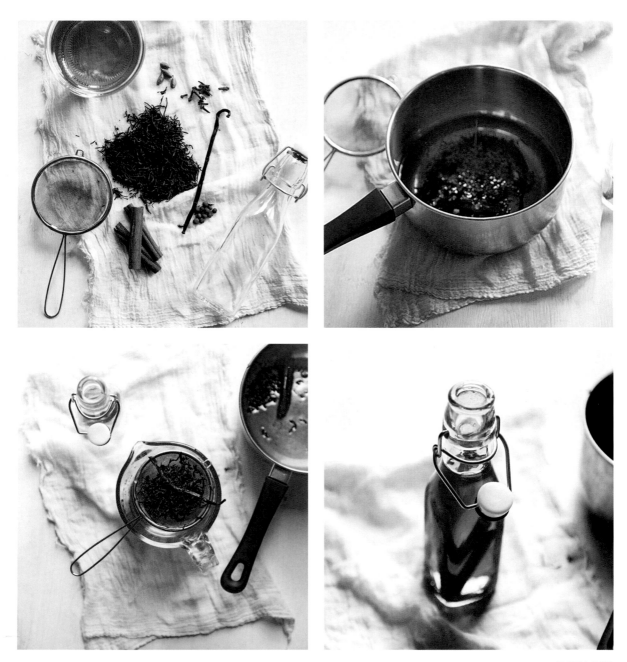

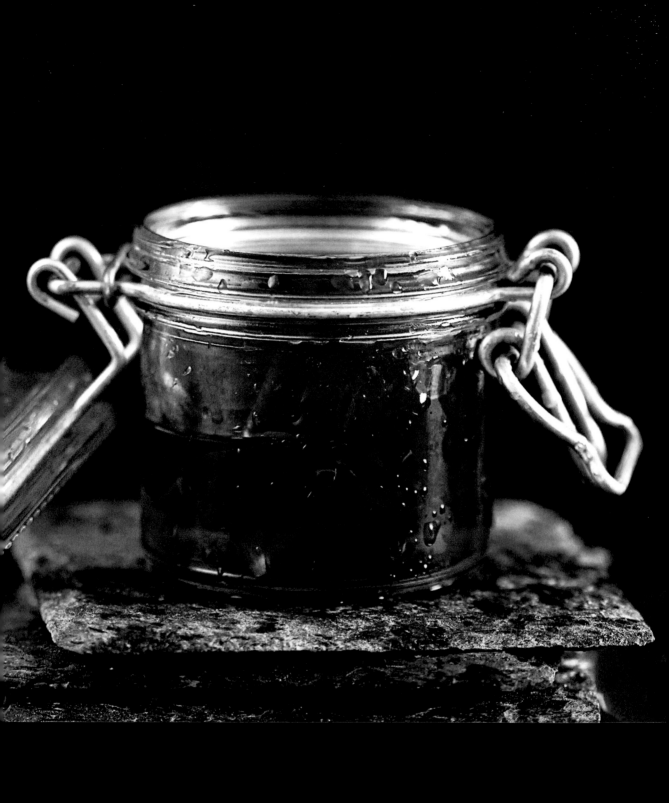

Rose-Almond Body Oil

You can harness the rays of the sun to infuse almond oil with rose petals, bottling up their aromatic and healing benefits all for yourself! The result is a pampering body oil that improves skin's texture and elasticity.

1 / Wash and dry a lidded jar that's large enough to fit the petals and oil. Make sure the jar and petals are completely dry to ensure that mold doesn't form.

2 / Measure and put the fresh rose petals in the jar and crush them up a bit with a spoon.

3 / Add the almond oil, completely covering the petals. You want the oil to reach at least 1 inch (2.5 cm) above the rose petals so they'll stay completely submerged even as they absorb the oil and swell.

4 / Seal the jar and keep it in a sunny place for between 7 and 10 days. Give it a shake every so often. After its time in the sun, strain the oil with cheesecloth, making sure to squeeze every bit of oil out of the roses.

5 / Transfer the oil to another jar with a lid, and apply liberally to your skin after showering.

MATERIALS	TOOLS	FREQUENCY OF USE
1 cup (16 g) fresh rose petals or dried roses	2 8-ounce (240-mL) lidded jars	**Daily**
1 cup (240 mL) sweet almond oil	Measuring cups	STORAGE ADVICE
	Spoon	**Use within 6 months**
	Cheesecloth	
	RECOMMENDED FOR	
	All skin types	

Cocoa-Rose Bath Salts

Soak away stress with bath salts suffused with the moisturizing power of cocoa butter and almond oil. Add dried roses and rose essential oil for an aromatherapy boost that eases tension and promotes relaxation.

1 / In a medium saucepan, bring 2 inches (5 cm) of water to a boil, and then reduce the heat to low.

2 / While the water is heating, measure the cocoa butter and drop it into a medium heat-safe glass bowl. Once the water is boiling, place the bowl inside the saucepan and melt the cocoa butter over low heat.

3 / Remove from heat and stir in the almond oil, then dump in the sea salt. Stir until the sea salt is evenly distributed throughout the cocoa butter and almond oil.

4 / Spread the resulting salt out on a cookie sheet and let the mixture air-dry for 24 hours.

5 / When the salt is dry, pour it into a jar with a lid. Add the dried rose petals, drizzle in the rose absolute essential oil with a pipette, and gently stir together. To enjoy, add ½ cup (130 g) salt to a warm bath.

MATERIALS	TOOLS	RECOMMENDED FOR
2 tablespoons cocoa butter	Medium saucepan	**All skin types**
2 tablespoons sweet almond oil	Measuring cups and spoons	FREQUENCY OF USE
2 cups (540 g) sea salt	Medium heat-safe glass bowl	**2 to 3 times per week**
¼ cup (4 g) dried rose petals	Spoon	STORAGE ADVICE
5 drops rose absolute essential oil	Cookie sheet	**Use within 6 months**
	8-ounce (240-mL) lidded jar	
	Pipette	

Pretty Packages
I love giving my homemade natural beauty indulgences as presents—and presenting them in clever containers too. For instance, try sharing the cocoa-rose bath salts (recipe on page 81) in these unexpected glass test tubes.

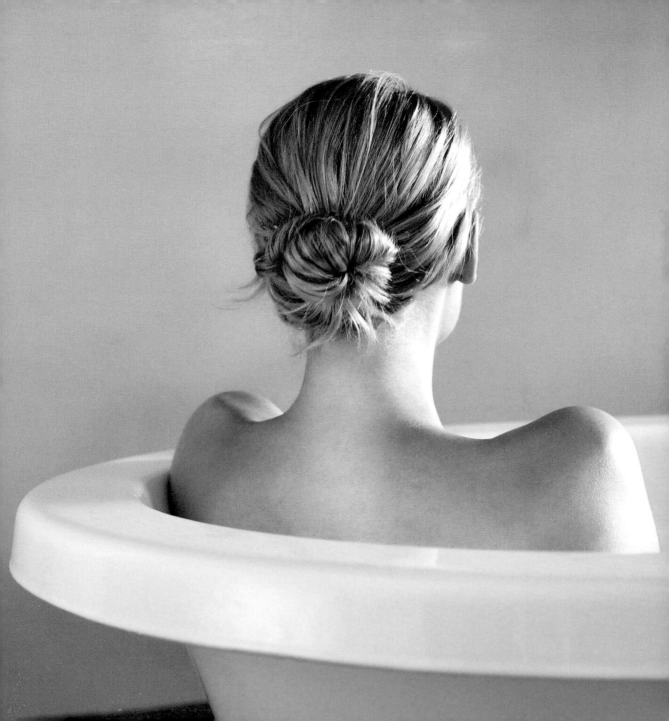

Lavender

It's no wonder that lavender is the most popular essential oil in the aromatherapy world. This calming mauve flower is both antiseptic and anti-inflammatory, and it offers a wealth of wonderful attributes—from toning skin and refreshing air to fighting insomnia and dandruff. But its true gift is its fragrance—just one whiff and you'll feel transported to Provence, France, where lavender fields in bloom make for an equally dreamy aroma and vista.

HONEY-LAVENDER BATH SOAK

3 tablespoons honey

13½-ounce (400-mL) can full-fat coconut milk

6 drops lavender essential oil

Whisk the honey with the coconut milk in a medium bowl, then add in the lavender essential oil with a pipette. Pour into a warm bath and soak it up.

LAVENDER-LEMONADE BODY SPRAY

½ cup (120 mL) orange flower water

1 tablespoon vodka

20 drops lemon essential oil

5 drops lavender essential oil

5 drops sandalwood essential oil

Pour the orange flower water and vodka into a 6-ounce (180-mL) spray bottle with a funnel, then use a pipette to drizzle in the lemon, lavender, and sandalwood essential oils. (Use a new bottle or one that's been sterilized, and be sure to label it—unless you like surprises!) Shake before each use and spray from head to toe.

AROMATIC HEADACHE SOOTHER

2 drops lavender essential oil

2 drops peppermint essential oil

1 teaspoon carrier oil (like sweet almond or grape-seed)

Using a pipette, drizzle the lavender and peppermint essential oils into the palm of your hand, then add the carrier oil. Rub the mixture into your temples, neck, and scalp to relieve tension headaches.

SOFTENING HAND SANITIZER

1 tablespoon witch hazel

2 tablespoons fresh aloe-vera gel

30 drops lavender essential oil

Mix the witch hazel and fresh aloe-vera gel in a 2-ounce (60-mL) bottle. Use a pipette to add the lavender essential oil, then cap and shake the container until the ingredients are well blended. Dispense a dime-size amount into your palm, and rub all over your hands and fingers to fight grime on the go. Carry everywhere!

Other Uses for Lavender

FALL-ASLEEP FACE MASK
Combine 1 teaspoon pulverized dried lavender with 1½ tablespoons honey. Apply to clean skin, avoiding the eyes. Leave it on for 15 minutes, then rinse off with warm water.

LAVENDER ICE FACE MASSAGE
Wrap a handful of ice cubes in a washcloth and sprinkle with 3 to 5 drops lavender essential oil. Gently massage your face and neck with it before bed. The massage and ice will help with fine lines and improve circulation.

LAVENDER LINEN SPRAY
With a funnel, pour 2 cups (470 mL) distilled water and 2 tablespoons vodka into a spray bottle. Use a pipette to add 15 to 20 drops lavender essential oil. Shake well and spritz linens or just around the room for a scent refresh.

DANDRUFF NIXER
To chase away flakes, massage 4 drops lavender essential oil into your scalp. Or add the essential oil to 1 cup (240 mL) warm water, if you prefer a hair rinse.

Revitalizing Herbal Detox Body Wrap

Applying a body mask is a bit more complicated than a plain old face mask, but the results—tighter, glowing skin all over—are way worth it! The clarifying essential oils, herbs, and clay in this wrap are excellent for toning the epidermis and stimulating your lymphatic system to remove toxins from the body.

1 / Measure and combine the thyme, rosemary, sage, and water in a small saucepan. Bring the water to a boil and remove from heat.

2 / Let the herbs infuse until the water is cool, about 30 minutes. Then filter out the herbs with a fine-mesh strainer. Reserve the water.

3 / Pour the infused water into a medium non-metal bowl. Add the clay with a non-metal measuring spoon, stirring until you have a smooth paste.

4 / Add the juniper and grapefruit essential oils with a pipette. Stir.

5 / To apply, first line a bathtub with a towel or sheet. Then spread the mask on your body and wrap each section with a piece of plastic wrap. Cover up using the towel or sheet, and relax in the tub for 20 to 30 minutes.

6 / Rinse off the mask in the shower and follow with a moisturizer.

Get All Wrapped Up

Body wraps are a highly relaxing way to remove toxins and excess fluids. All you need is a cotton bed sheet to re-create these expensive spa treatments at home.

SEAWEED This ocean botanical increases blood circulation and lymph flow, delivers vital minerals and vitamins, and improves skin texture. Mix 1 cup (110 g) seaweed powder with 3 tablespoons olive oil and enough water to make a spreadable paste. Using your hands, apply over the skin, starting from the feet and working up. Then wrap yourself up with a sheet.

MUD These masks, like clay masks, work by drawing out impurities and excess water while they dry on the skin. Use 1 cup (200 g) mineral-rich Dead Sea mud mixed with aloe-vera gel or oil. Apply by hand, and wrap up in a sheet.

CASTOR OIL This simple home remedy can help de-bloat, heal inflammation, improve circulation, make you more regular, and boost lymphatic function. Soak a scrap of flannel in 1 to 2 tablespoons castor oil, and place it over your abdomen or liver (just below your right breast). Cover the flannel with plastic wrap and hold a hot water bottle over it for up to 1 hour. Avoid if you're pregnant or menstruating.

MATERIALS

2 tablespoons fresh thyme

2 tablespoons fresh rosemary

2 tablespoons fresh sage

1 cup (240 mL) water

6 tablespoons French green clay

6 drops juniper essential oil

6 drops grapefruit essential oil

TOOLS

Measuring spoons

Small saucepan

Fine-mesh strainer

Medium non-metal bowl

Non-metal measuring spoon

Non-metal spoon

Pipette

Towel or sheet

Plastic wrap

RECOMMENDED FOR

All skin types

FREQUENCY OF USE

1 to 2 times per month

STORAGE ADVICE

Refrigerate covered and use within 7 to 10 days

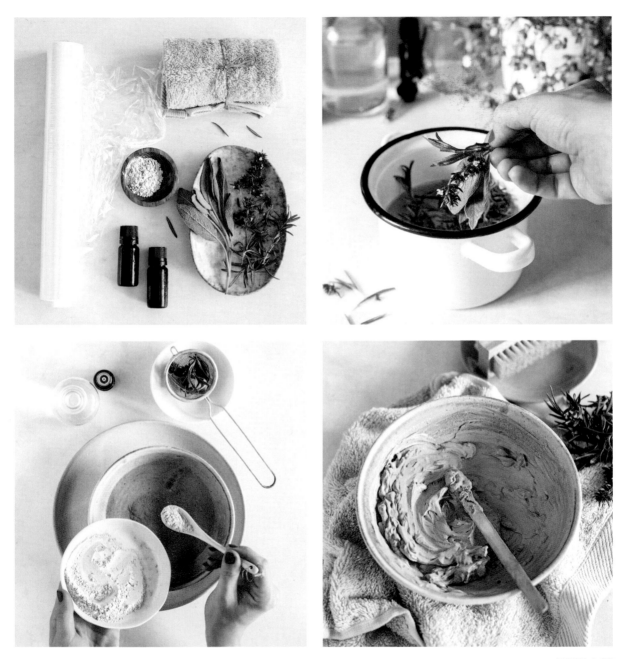

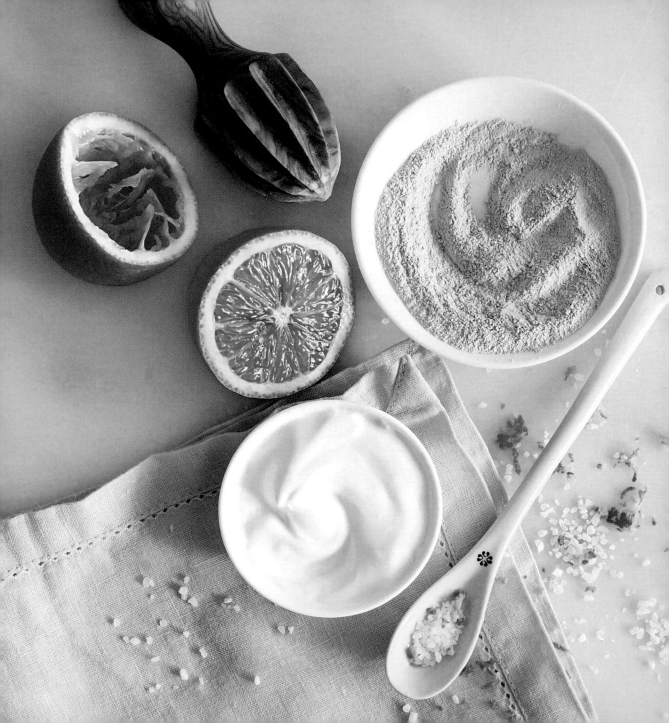

Cellulite-Smoothing Kiwi Scrub

Making a body scrub is simple—all you need is an oil and an exfoliant, like sugar or salt. Add in kiwi for its vitamins E and C (five times as much as an orange!), which together can help reduce the appearance of cellulite.

1 / Measure and pour the cane sugar into a small bowl.

2 / Peel one kiwi and add it to the bowl. Mash the fruit with the fork until it's coated with sugar.

3 / Measure and add the poppy seeds—which are fantastic for exfoliation!—and then stir with a spoon to combine the mixture.

4 / Slowly pour in the grape-seed oil and mix it well.

5 / Working in circular motions, apply the scrub in the shower with your hands, starting from the feet and moving upward.

6 / To extend this recipe's superpowers, use it as a mask after scrubbing it all over your body by leaving it on for 5 to 10 minutes. Then rinse with warm water and follow up with your favorite moisturizer.

MATERIALS	TOOLS	FREQUENCY OF USE
1 cup (250 g) cane sugar	**Measuring cups and spoons**	**Weekly**
1 kiwi	**Small bowl**	
2 tablespoons poppy seeds	**Fork**	STORAGE ADVICE
½ cup (120 mL) grape-seed oil	**Spoon**	**Refrigerate covered and use within 7 to 10 days**
	RECOMMENDED FOR	
	All skin types	

Citrus-Yogurt Bacne Banisher

Summer, sweat sessions, or hormonal changes can send your glands into overdrive, causing breakouts on your back and even derriere. Luckily, this scrub absorbs excess oil and eliminates pore-clogging dead skin cells.

1 / Use the zester to remove 1 tablespoon zest from 1 lemon, and then cut both lemons in half and juice them to extract ¼ cup (60 mL) juice.

2 / Mix the lemon juice, zest, and yogurt in a small bowl with a spoon. (Make sure these tools are plastic, wood, or ceramic instead of metal, which messes with the clay's benefits.)

3 / Add in the clay with a non-metal measuring spoon and stir until you have a smooth paste.

4 / Slowly add in the sea salt until you have a thick consistency that's still spreadable.

5 / Apply in the shower with a back scrubber, paying special attention to your back, upper arms, and bottom. Rinse with warm water and moisturize. Bye-bye, bacne!

MATERIALS	TOOLS	RECOMMENDED FOR
2 lemons	**Zester**	**Oily skin**
½ cup (125 g) organic, full-fat plain yogurt	**Knife**	
	Juicer	FREQUENCY OF USE
2 tablespoons bentonite clay	**Non-metal measuring cups and spoons**	**Weekly**
1 cup (270 g) sea salt	**Small non-metal bowl**	STORAGE ADVICE
	Non-metal spoon	**Use immediately**
	Back scrubber	

Raspberry-Basil Body Polish

You'll be tempted to eat this one, but resist! The ripe raspberries, honey, and brown sugar gently polish and revive dull areas of the body, while the basil adds a refreshing fragrance, purifies skin, and reduces redness.

1 / Combine the berries, basil, and honey in a blender. Pulse on low until you have a paste. (You can also use an immersion blender, if you happen to have one.)

2 / Transfer the mixture to a medium bowl and stir in the brown sugar with a spoon.

3 / Apply the scrub in the shower with your hands, working it in circular motions from your feet up. (If you like, you can also use this mixture as a mask by leaving it on the body for 5 to 10 minutes after you scrub with it.)

4 / Rinse with warm water and follow with moisturizer.

Tip / Sadly, it can't always be raspberry season. Fresh cranberries make a great substitute in winter.

MATERIALS	TOOLS	FREQUENCY OF USE
2 cups (250 g) raspberries	**Measuring cups**	**Weekly**
¼ cup (8 g) fresh basil	**Blender (or immersion blender)**	STORAGE ADVICE
¼ cup (90 g) honey	**Medium bowl**	**Refrigerate covered and use within 7 to 10 days**
1 cup (200 g) brown sugar	**Spoon**	
	RECOMMENDED FOR	
	All skin types	

Tropical Paradise Mango Scrub

Mangoes are a rich source of vitamin A, which sloughs off dead skin to reveal new, fresh cells underneath. And oats are also a fantastic exfoliator—especially for pesky rough patches on your elbows and knees.

1 / Use a knife to peel and cut the mango into cubes. Toss the cubes in a blender or food processor to purée, then transfer to a small bowl.

2 / Measure and add the oats and honey. Stir well with a spoon to combine.

3 / Apply the scrub in the shower with your hands, working in circular motions, starting at the feet and moving upward. (You can leave it on for 5 to 10 minutes to get the benefits of a mask too.)

4 / When you're finished with the scrub, wash it off with warm water. Apply your favorite moisturizer after you've stepped out of the shower.

MATERIALS	TOOLS	FREQUENCY OF USE
1 mango	**Knife**	**Weekly**
2 tablespoons oats	**Blender or food processor**	STORAGE ADVICE
1 teaspoon honey	**Small bowl**	**Best if used immediately**
	Measuring spoons	
	Spoon	
	RECOMMENDED FOR	
	Sensitive skin	

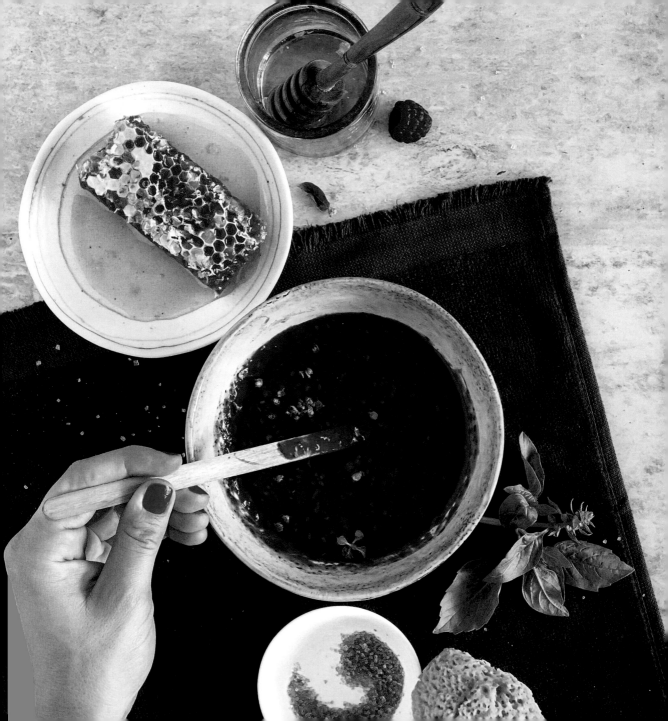

Charcoal to the Rescue

You can call on this little miracle worker in all kinds of situations.

WHITEN TEETH Open a capsule of activated charcoal into a cup. Add a tiny bit of water to make a paste, then dab onto your teeth. Wait 3 minutes and rinse.

EASE INDIGESTION Empty 2 charcoal capsules into a glass of water and drink 1 to 2 hours before or after meals.

TAKE THE STING OUT Mix 1 tablespoon activated charcoal powder and 1 tablespoon cornstarch with enough water to make a paste, then apply to a bug bite. Leave on for 15 minutes.

Charcoal+Tea-Tree Oil Detox Soaps

Activated charcoal soap cleanses, exfoliates, and clarifies—all without drying out the skin. It's particularly effective for people with acne-prone faces, as it gently removes dead epidermal cells and draws out the dirt, oil, and makeup that can clog pores. As for the tea-tree oil, it's a remarkable natural healer and does wonders for preventing and treating pimples.

1 / Using a knife, cut the shea-butter soap into 1-inch- (2.5-cm-) square chunks and put them in a heat-safe glass measuring cup.

2 / To melt the soap base, pour 2 inches (5 cm) of water into a small saucepan and place the measuring cup inside. Warm over medium-low heat on the stove top, stirring to break up the chunks. (Or heat it up in short bursts at 50-percent power in the microwave.) Be careful—it will be hot!

3 / Remove the measuring cup from the heat when the soap has almost melted. Stir it gently with a spoon to melt any remaining soap fragments.

4 / Open the activated charcoal capsules into the measuring cup and stir with a spoon to combine.

5 / Add in the tea-tree oil with a pipette. Stir together slowly to prevent the soap from forming bubbles.

6 / Select and ready your soap molds. Whatever containers you choose, spray them down with cooking spray and then wipe away any excess.

7 / Pour the soap mixture into the molds. Let them sit for 1 hour to completely set, then transfer the molds to the freezer for another hour or so.

8 / Remove the molds from the freezer—you should be able to pop your soaps right out.

9 / Use daily to wash your face and body, and watch those breakouts start to disappear!

MATERIALS	TOOLS	RECOMMENDED FOR	STORAGE ADVICE
¼ pound (125 g) melt-and-pour shea-butter soap base	Knife	**Oily skin**	**Use within 6 months**
5 activated charcoal capsules	Heat-safe glass measuring cup	**FREQUENCY OF USE**	
15 to 20 drops tea-tree oil	Small saucepan	**Daily**	
	Spoon		
	Pipette		
	Soap molds		
	Cooking spray		

PICK A MOLD, ANY MOLD

KITCHEN TOOLS You don't need fancy molds to make your own soap. A mini muffin tin is my favorite shape. Or try silicone baking molds.

REPURPOSED PACKAGING Use a plastic or cardboard container—hello, oatmeal canister!—as a mold, then slice the soap into bars when set.

Mustard-Ginger Bath Bombs

A hot bath is a great way to ease the ache when you're sick, and these bath bombs deliver more than a fun dose of fizz—although I do love that part! Plus, the mustard and ginger will have you sweating out the toxins.

1 / Stir the citric acid, cornstarch, baking soda, and ginger and mustard powders in a medium bowl. (Look for citric acid in the canning aisle of the grocery store.)

2 / Pour the sweet almond oil into a measuring cup. Add the eucalyptus essential oil with a pipette and stir.

3 / Pour the oil mixture into the bowl containing the dry ingredients and stir until you get a crumbly consistency.

4 / Use your hands to press the mixture into a mold. (Here, I used a muffin tin with cupcake liners.) Let sit in a cool spot overnight, then remove from the mold.

5 / To use, drop one bomb into a tub of warm water, hop in, and get your fizz fix for 20 minutes. Store the rest in a large plastic container for your next use.

MATERIALS	TOOLS	RECOMMENDED FOR
1 cup (240 g) citric acid	**Measuring cups and spoons**	**All skin types**
½ cup (60 g) cornstarch	**Spoon**	
1 cup (220 g) baking soda	**Medium bowl**	FREQUENCY OF USE
2 tablespoons powdered ginger	**Pipette**	**2 to 3 times per week**
2 tablespoons mustard powder	**Mold of your choosing**	
½ cup (120 mL) sweet almond oil	**2-quart (2-L) plastic container**	STORAGE ADVICE
20 drops eucalyptus essential oil		**Use within 6 months**

Cleopatra's Milk Bath

The Egyptian pharaoh was said to bathe in milk to keep her flesh soft and smooth—and if it's good enough for a queen, it's good enough for us. This bath is a lovely, soothing self-care ritual, especially after a long day.

1 / Pour the coconut milk into a medium bowl and stir to combine the liquid and coconut cream, if separated.

2 / Measure and drizzle in the honey. Stir until the mixture is nice and combined.

3 / Add the powdered milk, which is loaded with lactic acid that exfoliates and softens the skin—plus good fats that nourish. Stir to dissolve.

4 / Pour the mixture into the tub and bathe as usual. If saving some for later, transfer it to a container with a lid and refrigerate. Before using, let the mixture come to room temperature, then add to the bath.

Tip / Dealing with a skin rash or bug bites? Grind ½ cup (50 g) oats and add to reduce inflammation.

MATERIALS	TOOLS	STORAGE ADVICE
13½-ounce (400-mL) can full-fat coconut milk	**Medium bowl**	**Best if used immediately; refrigerate and use within 7 to 10 days**
¼ cup (90 g) honey	**Spoon**	
½ cup (60 g) full-fat powdered milk	**Measuring cup**	
	24-ounce (700-mL) lidded container	
	RECOMMENDED FOR	
	All skin types	
	FREQUENCY OF USE	
	As needed	

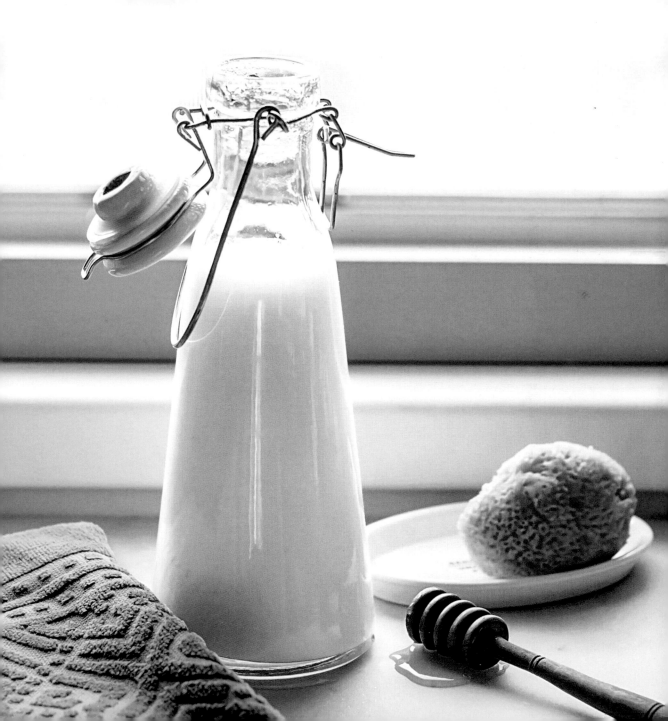

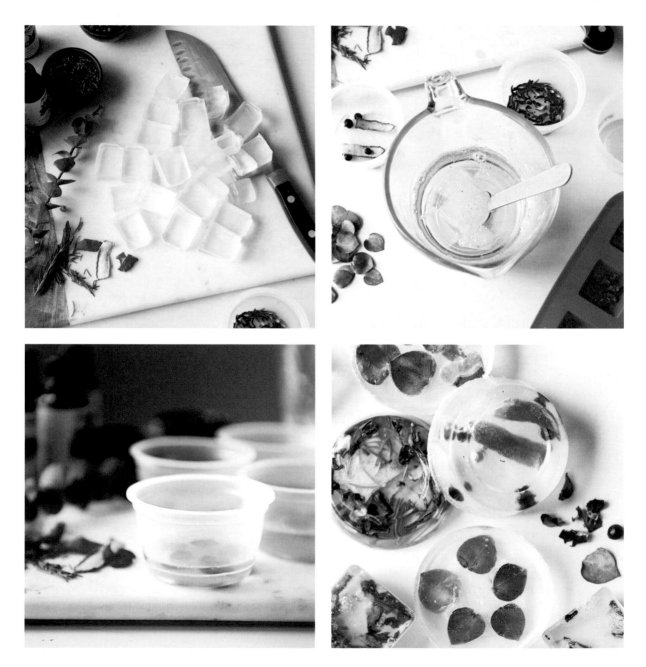

Pretty Herb + Spice Glycerin Soaps

If you've ever wanted to try making your own soap, take heart—it's easier than you ever could have imagined! Plus, melt-and-pour soaps allow for tons of customization. Experiment with your favorite herbs and spices for a truly personalized creation. These colorful soaps make lovely gifts for birthdays and holidays.

1 / Select your dried flowers, herbs, and spices—here, I used rosemary, eucalyptus, hibiscus, juniper berries, rose petals, and citrus peels, but anything goes with these sweet soaps. (Be aware, however, that some might change color—hibiscus turned blue, for instance. Hey, it's all an experiment!) Cut the botanicals into smaller pieces with a knife, if desired, and select the prettiest specimens. Set them aside.

2 / Cut the glycerin soap into 1-inch (2.5-cm) squares and put them in a heat-safe glass measuring cup. Pour 2 inches (5 cm) of water into a small saucepan, place the measuring cup inside, and warm over medium-low heat. (Or heat it up in short bursts at 50-percent power in the microwave.)

3 / Remove the measuring cup from the heat when the soap is soft. Stir to incorporate any soap fragments and break up any chunks.

4 / Let the soap cool slightly and then add your fragrances with a pipette. I suggest 5 drops per ounce (30 g) of soap used.

5 / Stir together slowly to prevent bubbles from forming. Gently tap the measuring cup on the countertop to release any larger trapped air bubbles.

6 / Time to select and prep your molds. This process gets messy, so you might want to repurpose something from the recycle bin, such as old milk cartons or yogurt cups. Mist the containers with cooking spray and wipe away any excess with a dishcloth.

7 / Arrange the dried botanicals in the bottom of your molds, then fill with the melted soap base.

8 / Let the soap set for 1 hour, then transfer the molds to the freezer for another hour. Take out the molds and bend to pop out the soap.

MATERIALS

½ cup (8 g) dried flowers, herbs, or spices of your choosing

1 pound (500 g) solid, clear glycerin soap base

2 complementary fragrance oils

TOOLS

Knife

Heat-safe glass measuring cup

Small saucepan

Spoon

Pipette

Soap molds

Cooking spray

RECOMMENDED FOR

All skin types

FREQUENCY OF USE

As needed

STORAGE ADVICE

Use within 6 months

MAKE IT YOUR OWN

FLOWER SOAPS Add dried flowers like chamomile, roses, calendula, or hibiscus.

TEA SOAPS Use your favorite teas, such as green, mint, or chai.

MOISTURIZING SOAPS For each 1 cup (300 g) soap, add 2 tablespoons of a moisturizing ingredient—like honey or aloe vera—or a mild oil, such as coconut.

EXFOLIATING SOAPS Add cornmeal, fresh coffee grounds, oats, or even sand for some nice scrub action.

Moisture-Boost Tangerine Body Wash

Packed with vitamin C, homemade citrus water energizes with its sunny fresh scent, while castile soap provides mellow sudsing power. Grab a pretty pump jar, and you'll be inventing reasons to get zestfully clean.

1 / Combine the water and tangerine peels in a small saucepan. Bring the water to a boil and then reduce the heat to medium for 5 minutes. Heat brings out the peels' natural oils, creating a distillation called a hydrosol.

2 / Remove the pan from the heat and let the water cool completely. Strain ½ cup (120 mL) of the water into a measuring cup and discard the lemon peels.

3 / Measure and add the castile soap, glycerin, and fractionated coconut oil. Stir to combine, then use a funnel to transfer the mixture to the container.

4 / Swirl the bottle to mix the ingredients. Pump into your hands, rub into a lather on your body, and rinse.

MATERIALS	TOOLS	RECOMMENDED FOR
1½ cups (360 mL) distilled water	Measuring cups and spoons	All skin types
2 tangerines	Small saucepan	
½ cup (120 mL) castile soap	Spoon	**FREQUENCY OF USE**
2 tablespoons vegetable glycerin	Funnel	As needed
2 tablespoons fractionated coconut oil	10-ounce (300-mL) pump bottle	**STORAGE ADVICE**
		Use within 3 months

Aromatic Jasmine-Aloe Shower Gel

This gentle, lightweight cleanser is perfect for those hot summer nights. Jasmine helps ease scars and stretch marks, and its fragrant scent makes for an intoxicating stress-buster. Mix with aloe vera for a skin-cooling treat.

1 / Bring the water to a boil and pour it over the jasmine tea bag. Steep for 5 minutes, then discard the tea bag and let the tea cool to room temperature.

2 / In a large measuring cup, combine the castile soap and aloe vera. Add ¼ cup (60 mL) of the jasmine tea to the soap-aloe mixture and stir—this 1:1 ratio of soap to liquid will suds up nicely but still be gentle on your skin.

3 / Measure and add the jojoba oil, then use a pipette to drizzle in the essential oil for a lovely floral aroma. Transfer the mixture to a bottle with a funnel.

4 / To use, swirl the bottle, disperse 2 to 3 pumps, and work into a lather all over your body. Rinse to finish.

MATERIALS	TOOLS	RECOMMENDED FOR
1 cup (240 mL) distilled water	Measuring cups and spoons	Normal to oily skin
1 jasmine tea bag	Spoon	
½ cup (120 mL) castile soap	Pipette	**FREQUENCY OF USE**
¼ cup (60 mL) fresh aloe-vera gel	10-ounce (300-mL) pump bottle	As needed
2 tablespoons jojoba oil	Funnel	**STORAGE ADVICE**
15 drops jasmine essential oil		Use within 3 months

Mind the Ratio

It helps to know how much liquid your container holds before you start. Fill your chosen container with water, then decant it into a measuring cup. Divide that measurement in half—that's the amount you need of both liquid and soap to create the 1:1 ratio required for your body wash.

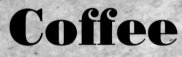

Coffee

Get ready for a new coffee addiction—turns out your morning brew is excellent for perking up skin. You can use coffee to attack cellulite, dark circles, and dryness, or embrace its diuretic powers to reduce swelling and puffiness in the a.m. Plus, this bean's antioxidants fight the free radicals that age skin. Now that's some coffee you should be happy to wake up and smell.

COFFEE CELLULITE SCRUB

½ cup (100 g) fresh coffee grounds
2 tablespoons brown sugar
¼ cup (60 mL) olive oil

Combine the coffee grounds and brown sugar in a small bowl. Apply the olive oil to any areas of your body that have cellulite, then rub the mixture into the oil in circular motions. Rinse off with warm water.

COFFEE-BANANA FOOT SCRUB

¼ cup (50 g) fresh coffee grounds
¼ cup (60 g) salt
¼ cup (60 mL) olive oil
½ banana

Combine the fresh coffee grounds, salt, olive oil, and ½ banana in a bowl. Then sit in an empty tub and slather the mixture all over your feet and lower legs. Let the mixture do its thing for 5 to 10 minutes. Give your feet and legs a really nice, long scrub, then rinse yourself (and the tub!) well.

COFFEE-INFUSED BODY OIL

1 cup (240 mL) sweet almond oil
½ cup (100 g) fresh coffee grounds

Place a small saucepan over a burner set to low heat. Put a heat-safe glass bowl inside the saucepan, pour in the almond oil and coffee grounds, and heat for 1 hour. Let cool, filter with a fine-mesh strainer, and transfer to a bottle with a funnel. Apply daily to diminish the appearance of cellulite.

DETOX COFFEE-GRAPEFRUIT BODY SCRUB

Drizzle of olive oil
½ ruby-red grapefruit
½ cup (100 g) fresh coffee grounds

Drip the olive oil on the cut side of the grapefruit, then dip the fruit into your coffee grounds. Apply the mixture to your body with the fruit, scrubbing in circular motions from your feet up. Add more olive oil and coffee grounds as needed.

Other Uses for Coffee

GREEK YOGURT–COFFEE MASK

Heat 1 tablespoon coconut oil in a saucepan or in the microwave for a few seconds to liquefy. Then combine with ¼ cup (70 g) organic, full-fat plain Greek yogurt, 2 tablespoons fresh coffee grounds, and juice from ½ lemon in a small bowl. Massage the mask onto your face and neck, and let it sit for 10 to 15 minutes. Rinse in the shower, exfoliating the skin gently while you remove the mask.

SKINNY BANANA-MOCHA SMOOTHIE

Put ½ cup (120 mL) cooled coffee, 1 banana, ½ cup (120 mL) unsweetened almond milk, 1 tablespoon unsweetened cocoa powder, 1 tablespoon almond butter, and a handful of ice cubes in a blender. Pulse until all the ingredients are smooth. Get your chocolate fix without excess calories!

COFFEE HAIR RINSE

Brew 1 cup (240 mL) coffee and allow it to cool to room temperature. Dilute it with 1 cup (240 mL) water and pour over your hair after shampooing. Leave for 5 minutes and then rinse to enrich the color of dark hair—and nix buildup and improve shine.

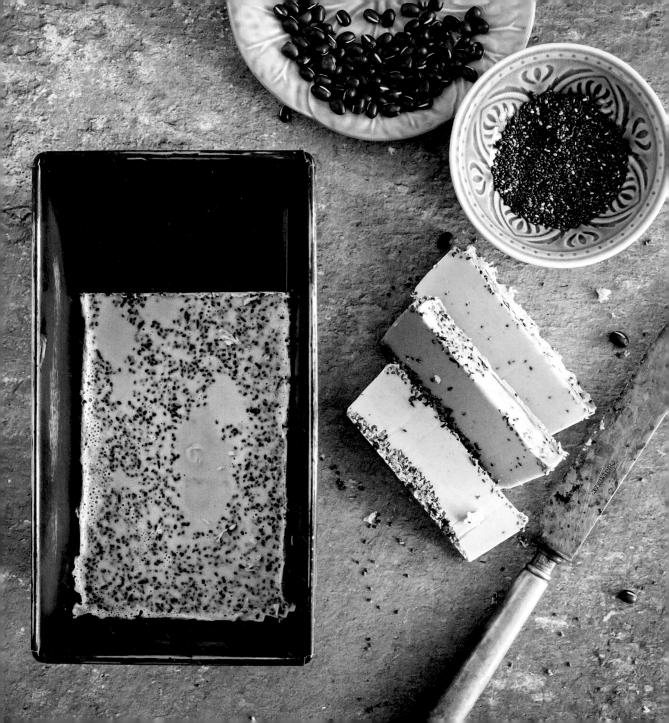

Seed+Bean Exfoliating Lotion Bars

This recipe combines the moisturizing benefits of a solid lotion bar with a powerful trio of skin-softening exfoliators. The gentle texture of ground beans, almonds, and chia seeds sloughs off dry flakes, while the cocoa and shea butters coat and protect skin. My favorite way to use it is in the shower—just rub the bar all over wet skin for a mess-free body buff!

1 / Measure the cocoa and shea butters. Mix them with a spoon in a medium heat-safe glass bowl.

2 / Bring 2 inches (5 cm) of water to a boil in a medium saucepan and reduce the heat to low. Place the glass bowl in your saucepan to melt the ingredients, then remove the bowl from the heat.

3 / Pulverize the almonds and adzuki beans in a coffee grinder.

4 / Add the chia seeds to the cocoa-shea butter mixture, followed by the ground almonds and adzuki beans. Stir until they're evenly distributed.

5 / Mist your chosen mold with cooking spray and wipe clean, then pour in the mixture and let cool. Once hard, pop the soaps out of the mold.

6 / To use, rub a bar all over your body in the shower to gently exfoliate.

Top Exfoliators

Dried beans and chia seeds might sound like unlikely ingredients for beauty recipes, but there's more than sugar and salt at your disposal for at-home exfoliation. You'll find plenty of face and body scrub options hiding in your pantry.

DRIED BEANS Adzuki beans are a Japanese red bean commonly used in Asian beauty routines. These finely ground beans often make an appearance in masks and cleansers for their exfoliating texture and natural saponin, which creates a foaming action.

ALMOND MEAL Finely ground almonds gently exfoliate, while their natural oils and fats moisturize and deliver vitamins A and E. Great for dry faces!

CHIA SEEDS In addition to its exfoliating abilities, this little superfood is packed with the omega-3 fatty acid alpha-lipoic acid, an antioxidant that fights free radicals and repairs damage.

CORNMEAL Much like oats, cornmeal is a great exfoliation choice for sensitive skin. Its fine texture softens in liquid so it gently removes dead skin and absorbs excess oil—all without irritating delicate skin.

MATERIALS	TOOLS	RECOMMENDED FOR	STORAGE ADVICE
½ cup (110 g) cocoa butter	Measuring cup	Dry skin	Use within 3 months
¼ cup (50 g) shea butter	Medium heat-safe glass bowl		
¼ cup (20 g) almonds	Spoon	FREQUENCY OF USE	
¼ cup (40 g) dry adzuki beans	Medium saucepan	As needed	
¼ cup (40 g) chia seeds	Coffee grinder		
	Soap mold		
	Cooking spray		

Mint-Mojito Foot Scrub

It's time to give your hardworking feet a little TLC with this invigorating foot scrub. Besides the refreshing, odor-masking scent, the mint helps reduce perspiration, while the salts exfoliate and improve circulation.

1 / Wash and zest the lime. Then use a knife to cut and juice it—you should have about 2 tablespoons.

2 / Chop up the fresh mint so you have 2 tablespoons. Pause to get a good whiff of that wonderful smell!

3 / Combine the lime juice, zest, and mint in a small bowl. Measure and add the sea and Epsom salts.

4 / If the coconut oil is solid, heat it up for a few seconds until it softens into a nice, buttery, workable texture. Add it to the bowl and stir to combine.

5 / To use, sit on the edge of the tub (use a large bowl if you don't have a tub) and thoroughly scrub your feet and calves. Let the scrub collect on the bottom of the tub as you massage the mixture over your skin.

6 / When you're done scrubbing, fill the tub or bowl with enough warm water to cover your feet. Soak for 10 to 15 minutes to pamper tired tootsies, then rinse.

MATERIALS	TOOLS	FREQUENCY OF USE
1 lime	Zester	**Weekly**
1 bunch fresh mint	Knife	
½ cup (130 g) sea salt	Measuring cups and spoons	STORAGE ADVICE
½ cup (120 g) Epsom salt	Small bowl	**Best if used immediately; refrigerate and use within 7 days**
2 tablespoons coconut oil	Spoon	
	Tub or large bowl	

RECOMMENDED FOR

All skin types

Banana-Honey Heel Softener

Our feet really take a beating—especially in summer, when all that strolling around in sandals can cause calluses and even cracked heels. This two-ingredient mask delivers major moisture—your feet will love it!

1 / Cut the banana in half and mash it in a small bowl with a spoon until the texture is nice and smooth.

2 / Measure and add the honey, stirring to combine.

3 / Apply to your feet while seated over the bathtub or a large bowl—it'll keep drips off your floor. Wrap each foot in plastic wrap after slathering the mask on.

4 / Relax for at least 10 minutes, then remove the plastic wrap and rinse off the banana. Your soles will be much softer!

5 / Now is a great time to follow with a scrub or pumice stone to exfoliate those stubborn calluses. Finish by massaging a rich moisturizer into your feet.

Tip / Before the mask, you can soak your feet for extra soothing. Add 1 cup (240 mL) white vinegar and ¼ cup (60 g) Epsom salt to a bowl of warm water. Soak your feet for 10 minutes to deodorize and soften your soles.

MATERIALS	TOOLS	RECOMMENDED FOR
1 banana	Knife	**All skin types**
1 teaspoon honey	Small bowl	
	Spoon	FREQUENCY OF USE
	Measuring spoon	**Weekly**
	Tub or large bowl	
	Plastic wrap	STORAGE ADVICE
	Pumice stone (optional)	**Use immediately**

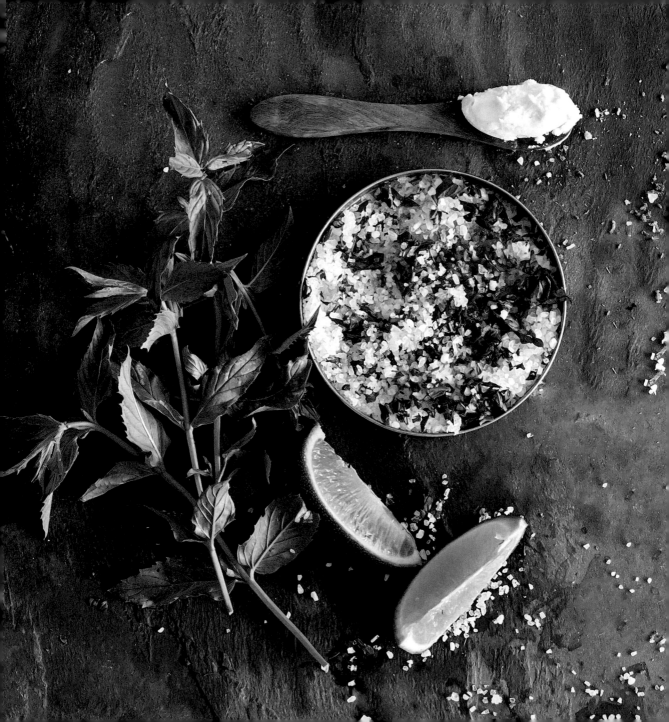

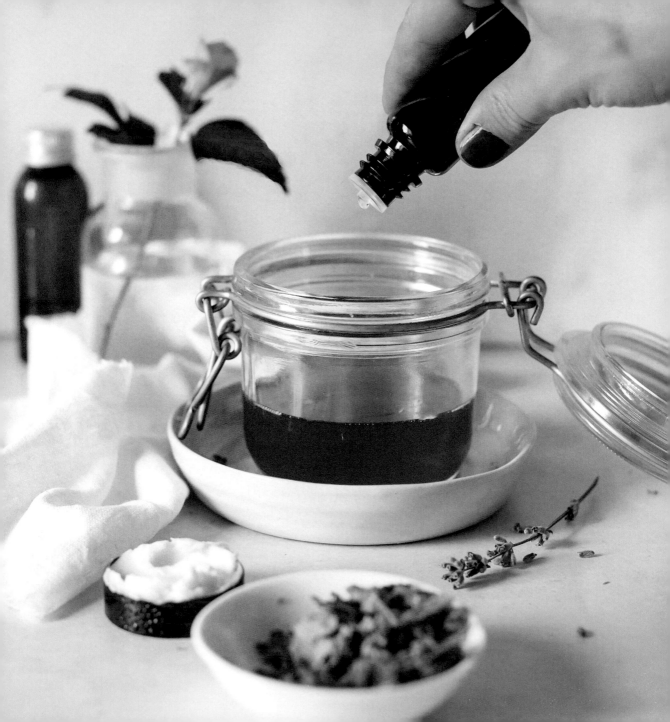

Comfrey + Olive Oil Hand Salve

This pretty purple flower has a long history in first aid—try it on a scrape sometime! And when its anti-inflammatory benefits merge with olive oil's moisturizing powers, you get a wonderfully soothing balm for dry hands.

1 / Measure the dried comfrey and add it to a clean, dry lidded jar. Pour in the olive oil, then replace the lid and shake the jar to completely coat the comfrey.

2 / Let the mixture sit in a sunny spot for 7 to 10 days. Give it a shake every so often. After its time in the sun, strain the comfrey out of the oil with cheesecloth.

3 / Measure out the shea butter and beeswax. Stir to combine them in a small heat-safe glass bowl.

4 / Bring 2 inches (5 cm) of water to a boil in a small saucepan, then reduce the heat to low. Place the glass bowl inside the saucepan and melt the ingredients.

5 / Remove the bowl from the heat. Stir in ½ cup (120 mL) of the comfrey-infused oil. (Save the leftovers for your next batch.) Add the lavender essential oil.

6 / Transfer to a container and let it sit until it's fully set. Replace the lid and keep your salve in a cool, dry spot.

MATERIALS	TOOLS	RECOMMENDED FOR
½ cup (16 g) dried comfrey leaves	Measuring cups and spoons	All skin types
1 cup (240 mL) olive oil	8-ounce (240-mL) lidded glass jar	**FREQUENCY OF USE**
2 tablespoons shea butter	Cheesecloth	As needed
2 tablespoons beeswax	Spoon	
10 drops lavender essential oil	Small heat-safe glass bowl	**STORAGE ADVICE**
	Small saucepan	Use within 6 months
	Pipette	
	6-ounce (180-mL) lidded container	

Rice-Parsley Spot Remover

When applying sunscreen, don't skip your hands; it'll lead to sun damage and dreaded dark spots. You can turn back the clock with this hand mask, which naturally lightens and exfoliates to reveal the fresh skin below.

1 / Measure and add the white rice to a bowl. Pour the distilled water over the rice and stir to combine.

2 / Let the mixture sit for at least 30 minutes and up to 2 hours—you want it to turn a milky white color. Then filter out the rice with a fine-mesh strainer and return the water to the bowl.

3 / Finely chop the parsley—its high levels of vitamins C and K give this recipe its spot-erasing superpowers—and add 1 cup (40 g) to the bowl, then measure and add the baking soda. Stir to combine all the ingredients.

4 / Transfer to a container with a lid and keep in the refrigerator. To use, apply a thick layer to the backs of your hands and let sit for 15 to 20 minutes. Gently massage when rinsing to exfoliate, then moisturize.

Tip / As a bonus, this mask can be applied to your face, neck, and chest, too!

MATERIALS	TOOLS	RECOMMENDED FOR
¼ cup (60 g) uncooked white rice	Measuring cups and spoons	All skin types
½ cup (120 mL) distilled water	Small bowl	**FREQUENCY OF USE**
1 bunch parsley	Spoon	2 to 3 times per week
1 tablespoon baking soda	Fine-mesh strainer	
	Knife	**STORAGE ADVICE**
	12-ounce (350-mL) lidded container	Refrigerate and use within 14 days

Perfect-for-Your-Purse Solid Perfume

Playing scent mixologist is just plain fun. Try a blend of top notes (palmarosa, lemongrass, lavender), bright middle notes (jasmine, neroli, Mandarin orange), and lingering base notes (vetiver, sandalwood, frankincense).

1 / Measure out the jojoba oil and beeswax. Combine them in a small heat-safe glass bowl with a spoon.

2 / Pour 2 inches (5 cm) of water into a small saucepan and bring to a boil, then lower the heat and put the bowl in the saucepan to melt the oil and beeswax.

3 / Remove from heat. Add the grapefruit, sweet orange, peppermint, and lemongrass essential oils with a pipette.

4 / Stir to combine, then pour the mixture into the small container and let it harden. Store in a cool, dry place.

5 / To apply, rub a small amount on your wrists or behind your ears.

MATERIALS	TOOLS	RECOMMENDED FOR
3 teaspoons jojoba oil	Measuring spoon	All skin types
¾ teaspoon beeswax	Small heat-safe glass bowl	**FREQUENCY OF USE**
3 drops grapefruit essential oil	Spoon	As needed
2 drops sweet orange essential oil	Small saucepan	**STORAGE ADVICE**
2 drops peppermint essential oil	Pipette	Use within 2 months
1 drop lemongrass essential oil	2-ounce (60-mL) lidded container	

Fresh + Sweet Customizable Scented Oil

Think about your best scent memories—a whiff of citrus may remind you of innocent summers, while vanilla may conjure up more sensual moments. Customize your perfume with aromas you love to boost your mood.

1 / Measure out the grape-seed or jojoba oil. Use a funnel to pour it into an amber bottle with either a spray or roll-on top.

2 / With a pipette, drizzle in the vanilla, lavender, and peppermint essential oils, then gently shake the mixture to distribute the ingredients.

3 / To use, spritz lightly or roll onto your wrists and other pulse points.

Tip / Storing your perfume oil in an amber bottle will prevent the essential oils from degrading—so your scent will stay stronger longer!

MATERIALS	TOOLS	FREQUENCY OF USE
2 tablespoons grape-seed or jojoba oil	Measuring spoons	Daily
6 drops vanilla essential oil	Funnel	**STORAGE ADVICE**
5 drops lavender essential oil	1-ounce (30-mL) amber bottle with spray or roll-on top	Use within 2 months
1 drop peppermint essential oil	Pipette	
	RECOMMENDED FOR	
	All skin types	

Roll On Sweetness

Try one of the following essential oil combinations in an aromatherapy roll-on.

STRESS 6 drops clary sage, 4 drops lavender, 2 drops lemon

SORE MUSCLES 2 drops ginger, 1 drop black pepper, 4 drops peppermint, 5 drops eucalyptus

WINTER BLUES 8 drops orange, 2 drops ylang ylang

CONCENTRATION 6 drops rosemary, 4 drops lemon, 2 drops peppermint

SLEEP 7 drops Roman chamomile, 5 drops lavender

Coconut Oil

This super ingredient is my absolute favorite. One of the most versatile natural beauty products around, coconut oil has a scent that conjures up a relaxing day by the ocean, but it also conditions and nourishes skin and hair like nothing else! It's naturally antifungal, too, making it a soothing moisturizer to use from head to toe. Stock some in your pantry, and all the benefits of a beach vacation will never be more than a jar away.

WHIPPED BODY LOTION

½ cup (110 g) shea butter
¼ cup (50 g) coconut oil

Pour 2 inches (5 cm) of water into a small saucepan and place a small heat-safe glass bowl on top. Melt the shea butter and coconut oil in the bowl, then refrigerate for 1 hour. Beat the ingredients with a hand mixer on medium for 5 to 7 minutes or until they fluff up, using a rubber spatula to scrape down the sides of the bowl. Transfer the body butter to a 6-ounce (180-mL) lidded glass container and enjoy for up to 6 months.

SOFTENING DETOX BATH

¼ to ½ cup (50–100 g) coconut oil
2 cups (480 g) Epsom salt

Combine a big scoop of coconut oil and Epsom salt, and add to a warm bath. While the salt detoxes your skin, the oil will coat and hydrate your body for a silky-smooth feel. Apply more oil post-bath so you can go to bed all warm and velvety to the touch!

COCONUT OIL SHAVING CREAM

¼ cup (50 g) coconut oil
½ cup (120 mL) fresh aloe-vera gel
4 to 6 drops lavender essential oil

Melt the coconut oil and combine it with the fresh aloe-vera gel and lavender essential oil. Stir together and store in a 6-ounce (180-mL) plastic container. When ready to apply, spread a thin layer on your skin and let sit a couple of minutes before shaving. The aloe will soften your follicles for an easier shave, while the coconut oil will moisturize the skin, helping to prevent razor burn and skin irritation.

MINTY COCONUT TOOTHPASTE

3 tablespoons coconut oil
3 tablespoons baking soda
10 to 15 drops peppermint essential oil
Stevia to taste (optional)

Warm the coconut oil in a small saucepan or the microwave until it's liquefied, if needed. Stir in the baking soda and peppermint essential oil, and store in a 3-ounce (90-mL) sealed container. (Don't like the taste? Add a bit of stevia, a natural sweetener.)

Other Uses for Coconut Oil

STRETCH MARK LOTION

Mix ½ cup (100 g) coconut oil with 15 drops grapefruit essential oil in a small bowl. Stir to combine, then store in a 4-ounce (120-mL) lidded container. Apply daily to your skin to help stave off stretch marks.

CUTICLE AND HAND MOISTURIZER

Massage 1 teaspoon coconut oil into your nail beds for a simple cuticle cream that also helps strengthen nails. While you're at it, rub the oil over the rest of your hands—it will also aid in reducing fine lines and age spots.

COCONUT MAKEUP REMOVER PADS

Dab a cotton pad with ½ teaspoon coconut oil for a chemical-free eye makeup remover that cleanses and moisturizes all in one. To use, gently wipe over your eye area. That's it!

COCONUT CONDITIONING HAIRSPRAY

Mix 2 cups (470 mL) distilled water with 2 tablespoons fractionated coconut oil (which stays liquid without separating). Funnel the mix into a 24-ounce (710-mL) spray bottle, then add 5 drops rosemary essential oil with a pipette. Spritz on whenever you need extra moisture.

DIY Probiotic Deodorant

You may be thinking, "DIY deodorant? No way!" But it's easy to make and surprisingly effective. Say good-bye to the chemicals in commercial deodorants—this formula will have your pits fresher and softer than ever.

1 / Measure out the coconut oil and shea butter, then combine them in a small heat-safe glass bowl.

2 / Boil 2 inches (5 cm) of water in a small saucepan, then turn the heat to low. Put the bowl in the saucepan and let the coconut oil and shea butter melt and mingle.

3 / Take the bowl off the heat and let it cool for a few minutes. Add the cornstarch, kaolin clay, probiotic-powder capsules, and vitamin E capsules. Drizzle in the lavender essential and tea-tree oils with a pipette.

4 / Stir, then transfer to a lidded container and let it set. Add the lid and stash in a cool, dry spot. To use, apply to clean, dry armpits. Reapply after exercise or as needed.

MATERIALS	TOOLS	RECOMMENDED FOR
3 tablespoons coconut oil	Non-metal measuring cups and spoons	All skin types
2 tablespoons shea butter	Small heat-safe glass bowl	FREQUENCY OF USE
¼ cup (30 g) cornstarch	Small saucepan	Daily
¼ cup (40 g) kaolin clay	Pipette	
3 probiotic-powder capsules	Non-metal spoon	STORAGE ADVICE
3 vitamin E capsules	6-ounce (180-mL) lidded container	Use within 3 months
10 drops lavender essential oil		
10 drops tea-tree oil		

Zinc-Coconut Sunscreen

Long worn for sun protection (remember those white noses?), the mineral zinc oxide reflects and absorbs UVA and UVB rays so your skin doesn't have to. Use non-nano uncoated zinc oxide for optimum coverage.

1 / Measure the coconut oil, shea butter, and beeswax, and stir them in a small heat-safe glass bowl.

2 / Bring 2 inches (5 cm) of water to a boil in a small saucepan, then reduce the heat to low. Place the glass bowl in the saucepan and melt the ingredients together.

3 / Remove from heat and let cool for a few minutes. Add the red raspberry-seed oil and vitamin E capsules, and drizzle in the carrot-seed oil with a pipette. (These oils offer natural SPF protection.) Add the zinc oxide last, covering your nose and mouth when handling.

4 / Transfer the mix to a container and let it sit until fully hardened. Replace the lid and keep in a cool, dry spot.

MATERIALS	TOOLS	RECOMMENDED FOR
1 cup (200 g) coconut oil	Measuring cups and spoons	All skin types
2 tablespoons shea butter	Spoon	FREQUENCY OF USE
¼ cup (60 g) beeswax	Small heat-safe glass bowl	As needed
2 tablespoons red raspberry-seed oil	Small saucepan	
10 vitamin E capsules	Pipette	STORAGE ADVICE
20 drops carrot-seed oil	16-ounce (470-mL) lidded container	Use within 6 months
2 tablespoons non-nano uncoated zinc oxide		

Sunscreen Savvy

Be aware that this deliciously scented coconut sunscreen isn't hardy enough for all-day wear in strong sun—it's about SPF 20. To use, rub it on 15 minutes before you head outside and reapply every 2 hours—or every time you hit the pool or the waves!

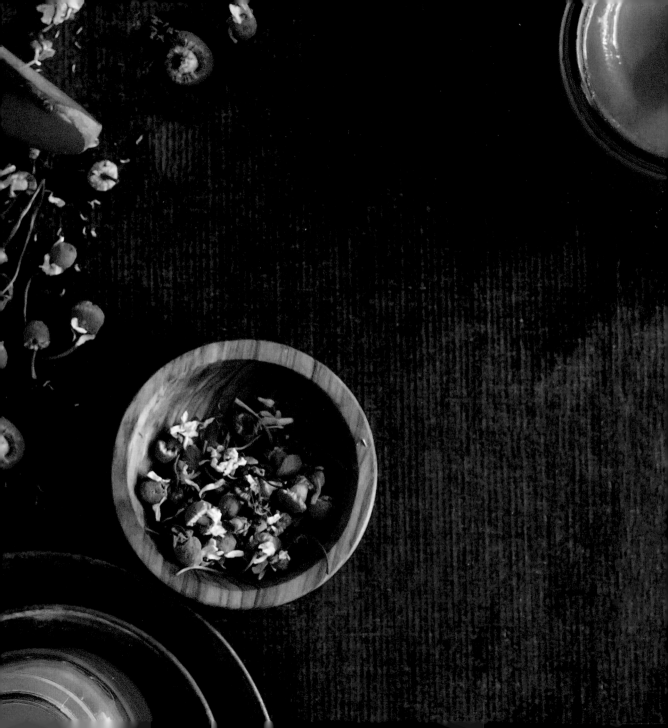

HAIR

The elusive good hair day can
be yours for keeps with this
arsenal of shampoos, masks,
scalp scrubs, and sprays.
Go ahead, let your hair down!

HAIRCARE BASICS

Everyone's hair is different, but whether your locks are superfine and oily (like mine) or dry and coarse, your mane will definitely benefit from these healthy hair habits. It might require a period of adjustment to train your tresses or reverse the damage from too much sun or styling, but this simple system will keep your hair strong, shiny, and soft—you won't be able to stop running your fingers through it, I promise.

DAILY

Eat Right If you experience hair breakage, slow growth, or hair loss, look for a supplement with vitamin B (biotin), zinc, and iron. Adding more omega-3s to your diet will also keep your hair in tip-top shape—good food sources include flaxseeds, chia seeds, walnuts, fish, and fish oil.

TWICE A WEEK

1 / Shampoo How often you wash your hair is a matter of preference, but you should aim to clean it every 2 to 3 days. (Some hair types, like fine or oily, might need more frequent sudsing.) Go with a gentle shampoo that doesn't strip away your hair's natural oils, then slowly lengthen the time between washings to give your hair a chance to regulate itself. When shampooing, concentrate the suds at the back of your crown, and don't fret about the ends—rinsing carries the shampoo all the way down the strand.

2 / Condition If your hair is dry or damaged, apply a conditioner after each shampoo session to moisturize, soften, and smooth your locks. Work it all over your hair, focusing on the ends, but avoid the scalp if your hair is fine or oily. Let it soak for 3 minutes (shave your legs while you wait!), then rinse.

3 / Rinse I love herbal hair rinses! (In fact, some people with more oily scalps forgo conditioners and follow up shampooing with this simple treatment instead.) They're especially great for normal or oily hair that doesn't need a cream conditioner after each shampoo. Use a rinse with herbs and diluted apple-cider vinegar to balance your hair's pH level, remove product buildup, and create shine.

4 / Brush and Style How you brush, dry, and style your hair can have a big impact on its health. Keep frizz and breakage to a minimum by using gentle, natural bristles in your combs and brushes. Give your hair a break from the drying, damaging effects of hairdryers, curling irons, and straighteners whenever possible. And when you do use heated hair tools, avoid their hottest settings.

WEEKLY

Apply a Hair Mask I prefer a weekly hair mask or oil treatment instead of conditioning after each shampoo. Use rich, natural oils like argan and coconut to nourish and repair hair. Masks are usually applied to dry locks and then left on for at least 30 minutes. You can add heat by warming the oils before applying them, or try a shower cap or towel to intensify the conditioning. Remove the mask with shampoo and follow with a hair rinse to nix any lingering residue.

Show Your Scalp Some Love Keeping your scalp in good condition will maintain your hair's health and help it grow faster. Why? Because it's where the follicles are—aka, where hair gets started. Give yourself regular scalp massages to increase circulation, and try a scrub to exfoliate, stimulate growth, and remove product buildup.

EVERY 6 TO 8 WEEKS

Get Frequent Haircuts Regular trims encourage new hair growth and remove any split ends.

DAMAGED + DRY HAIR

Battling frizz or split ends? Your hair needs moisture. Drench the roots with nutrient-rich conditioning oils, and choose repairing botanicals and essential oils that coat the hair shaft.

CONDITIONERS

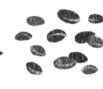

Shea Butter

Argan Oil

BOTANICALS

Sage
(dark hair)

Chamomile
(light hair)

ESSENTIAL OILS

Sandalwood

Geranium

OILY HAIR

Avoid overwashing, stick with lightweight conditioners that won't add even more oil, and go for plants and essential oils that cut grease and regulate the scalp's oil production.

CONDITIONERS

Neem Oil

Aloe Vera

BOTANICALS

Peppermint

Thyme

ESSENTIAL OILS

Cedarwood

Lemon

NORMAL + FINE HAIR

It's challenging to soften and smooth normal or fine hair without weighing it down. Skip heavy products, and look for ingredients like rosemary and nettle that nourish and strengthen hair.

CONDITIONERS

Jojoba Oil

Coconut Milk

BOTANICALS

Oat Straw

Nettle

ESSENTIAL OILS

Rosemary

Lavender

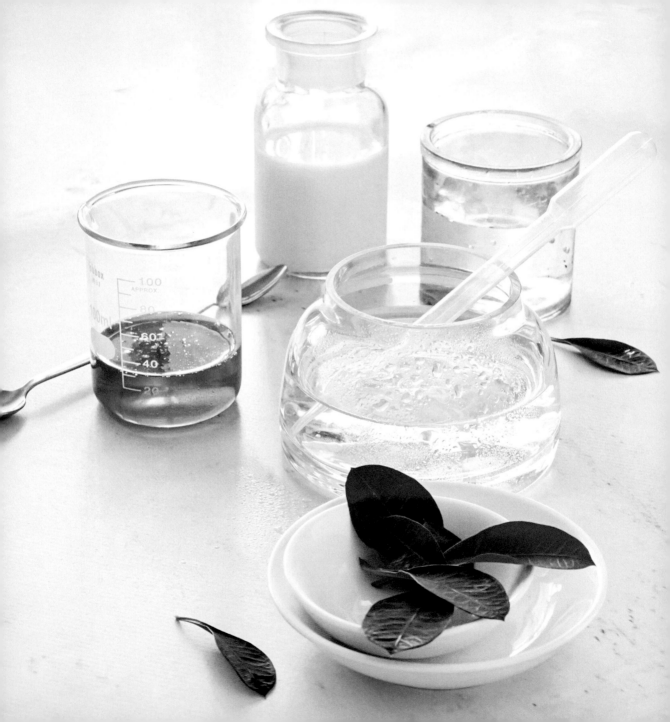

Tea-Tree Oil Dandruff Shampoo

Dandruff is one of the most vexing hair issues—have you ever worn a black shirt, only to spend the whole day worried that everyone could spot those telltale white flakes? But there's no need for harsh medicated shampoos. This gentle one gets it done with coconut milk and jojoba oil (which nourish dry scalps) and naturally antifungal, flake-fighting tea-tree oil.

1 / Measure and mix the coconut milk, castile soap, and glycerin in a large measuring cup. Stir with a spoon.

2 / Follow up with the jojoba oil, then use a pipette to drizzle in the tea-tree oil. With a spoon, mix well to combine all the ingredients.

3 / Use a funnel to pour the mixture into a bottle with a hand pump or a dispenser cap.

4 / Swirl to redistribute the oils before each use. Condition after shampooing.

Tip / You can also massage tea-tree oil right into your scalp to scare off dandruff. Combine 10 drops with 2 tablespoons of a carrier oil—like olive or jojoba—and apply it to your scalp. Leave on overnight and shampoo out in the morning.

Boost Your Shampoo

Not ready to DIY your own shampoo? Just switch to a gentle natural shampoo and customize it to meet your specific hair needs.

DRY HAIR Add 1 tablespoon nourishing jojoba or olive oil to an 8-ounce (240-mL) bottle of shampoo and shake.

OILY HAIR Bentonite clay is a great addition if you have an oily scalp. Add 1 tablespoon to your usual shampoo and agitate.

HAIR LOSS Castor oil has long been touted as a natural solution for stopping hair loss in its tracks and stimulating hair growth. Add 1 to 2 tablespoons to an 8-ounce (240-mL) shampoo bottle. Massage into your scalp each use.

PRODUCT BUILDUP Combine a dollop of shampoo with 1 teaspoon baking soda in your hand, and you've got a simple clarifying shampoo that strips away the chemicals and residue that your styling products leave behind.

VOLUME Adding salt to your shampoo is an easy trick for volumizing hair. In your palm, combine equal parts shampoo and kosher salt, and wash normally.

MATERIALS	TOOLS	RECOMMENDED FOR	STORAGE ADVICE
¼ cup (60 mL) coconut milk	Measuring cups and spoons	Normal to oily hair	Refrigerate and use within 1 month
½ cup (120 mL) liquid castile soap	Spoon		
1 tablespoon vegetable glycerin	Pipette	**FREQUENCY OF USE**	
2 teaspoons jojoba oil	Funnel	2 to 3 times per week	
10 drops tea-tree oil	8-ounce (240-mL) bottle with a hand pump or dispenser cap		

Customizable Dry Shampoo

Raid your pantry for simple ingredients to make your own dry shampoo, which is a life-saver for touching up dirty hair or making a great style last just one more day. Plus, these recipes enhance your natural color.

1 / Choose a recipe for your hair (see Materials, below).

2 / Measure and pulverize the oats in a coffee grinder until it's a fine powder. Combine the oat powder with the dry ingredients specified for your hair color in a small bowl. Mix thoroughly with a spoon.

3 / Use a pipette to drizzle in the suggested essential oil. Stir, then pour the mixture into an empty spice container. (Make sure to label it!)

4 / Shake the bottle before each use, then sprinkle the powder onto the roots of dry hair to absorb excess oil. Brush the dry shampoo through your locks, or use a hairdryer and your fingers to work it through your roots.

MATERIALS

1 tablespoon oats

FOR LIGHT HAIR

¼ cup (30 g) cornstarch

10 drops chamomile essential oil

FOR DARK HAIR

2 tablespoons cornstarch

2 tablespoons unsweetened cocoa powder

½ teaspoon cinnamon

10 drops lavender essential oil

TOOLS

Measuring cups and spoons

Coffee grinder

Small bowl

Spoon

Pipette

6-ounce (180-mL) spice container

RECOMMENDED FOR

All hair types

FREQUENCY OF USE

As needed

STORAGE ADVICE

Use within 6 months

Second-Day Reset Spray

Sudsing up daily can create both dry strands and oily roots, leading to a vicious cycle of overwashing. This spray is your secret weapon when training tresses to need fewer shampoo sessions—it gives a nice volume boost too!

1 / Measure and combine the witch hazel, distilled water, and vodka in a large measuring cup. Use a pipette to drizzle in the essential oil of your choosing.

2 / Add the cornstarch (with the cocoa powder, if you have dark hair). Stir with a spoon.

3 / Using a funnel, pour the liquid into a spray bottle. Just don't use a fine-mist spray bottle—it will clog easily.

4 / To use, shake and hold the bottle 2 inches (5 cm) from your roots, then spritz. Style with a hairdryer.

Tip / Cornstarch and vodka can dry out the scalp, but luckily the witch hazel in this recipe counteracts them! Look for a witch hazel that doesn't contain alcohol.

MATERIALS

¼ cup (60 mL) witch hazel

¼ cup (60 mL) distilled water

2 tablespoons vodka

5 drops essential oil (like lavender or rosemary)

FOR LIGHT HAIR

2 tablespoons cornstarch

FOR DARK HAIR

2 tablespoons cornstarch

1 tablespoon unsweetened cocoa powder

TOOLS

Measuring cup and spoons

Pipette

Spoon

Funnel

6-ounce (180-mL) spray bottle

RECOMMENDED FOR

Normal to oily hair

FREQUENCY OF USE

As needed

STORAGE ADVICE

Use within 2 months

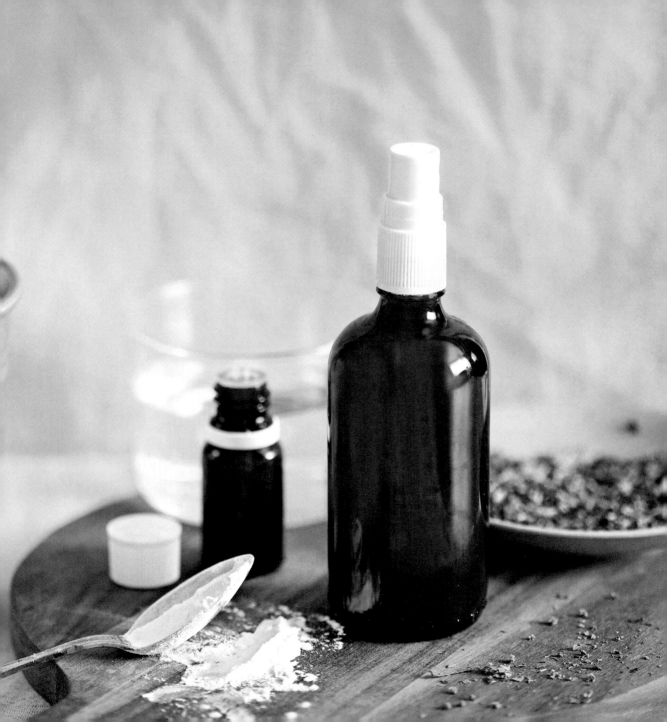

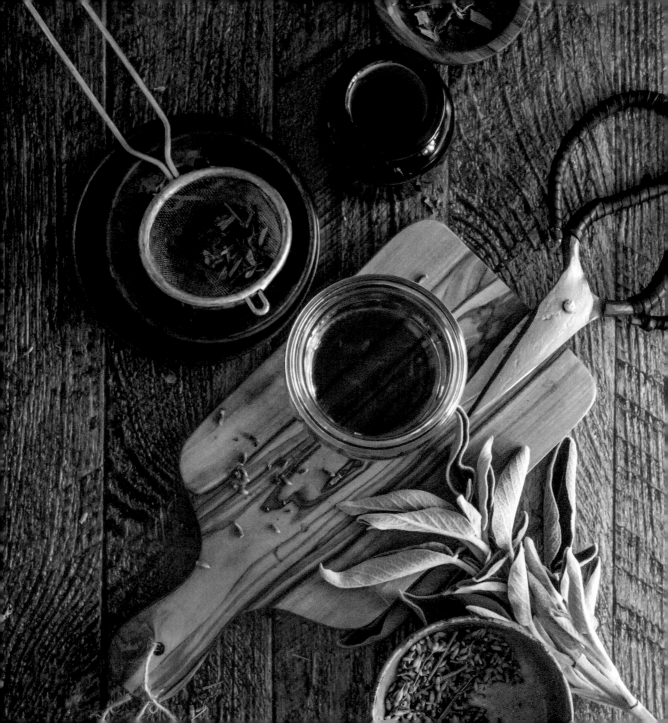

Rosemary-Nettle Rinse

Soothe your scalp, encourage follicle growth, and make your locks oh-so-touchable with this fragrant infusion. For a sweet addition, pour on the apple juice—it'll help restore your scalp's natural pH levels.

1 / Measure the water and bring to a boil in the small saucepan, then remove from heat and pour over the nettle and rosemary. (I use a French press for this step, but a plain old bowl works.) Cover and let steep until the liquid cools to room temperature (about 10 minutes).

2 / Use the fine-mesh strainer to filter out the herbs, retaining as much liquid as possible. With a funnel, pour the liquid into a bottle, then add the apple juice.

3 / To use, shampoo and then pour 1 cup (240 mL) of the rinse over your head. (If you're using a spray bottle, spritz to fully saturate.) Comb through your hair and leave it in, then dry and style as usual.

Tip / Light-haired ladies, try dried chamomile instead of rosemary—it'll help keep your blonde color bright.

MATERIALS	TOOLS	RECOMMENDED FOR
2 cups (470 mL) distilled water	Measuring cups and spoons	Dry hair or scalp
2 tablespoons dried nettle	Small saucepan	FREQUENCY OF USE
2 tablespoons dried rosemary	French press or medium bowl	2 to 3 times per week
¼ cup (60 mL) unsweetened apple juice	Fine-mesh strainer	
	Funnel	STORAGE ADVICE
	24-ounce (710-mL) squeeze or spray bottle	Refrigerate and use within 1 month

Herbal Buildup Remover

Apple-cider vinegar is a hair wonder—it smooths the cuticle to create loads of shine and removes buildup on the shaft for a major boost in volume. Plus, the lavender and sage in this recipe combat excess oil and dandruff.

1 / Bring the water to a boil in the small saucepan. Take it off the burner, then douse the sage and lavender with the liquid in a French press or bowl. Let them steep for at least 30 minutes—add time for a stronger treatment.

2 / Remove the herbs with a fine-mesh strainer, then discard the solids and pour the liquid into a spray bottle with a funnel. Add the apple-cider vinegar and shake.

3 / To use, spray or pour the rinse all over your hair after shampooing. Massage into your scalp and comb through the ends of your hair.

4 / Let the solution sit for a few minutes and then wash it out with warm water. For a more potent effect, you can forgo the final rinse. (Don't worry—you won't end up smelling like vinegar!)

MATERIALS	TOOLS	RECOMMENDED FOR
3 cups (710 mL) distilled water	Measuring cups and spoons	Normal to oily hair
¼ cup (8 g) dried sage	Small saucepan	FREQUENCY OF USE
¼ cup (10 g) dried lavender	French press or medium bowl	2 to 3 times per week
3 tablespoons apple-cider vinegar	Fine-mesh strainer	
	32-ounce (950-mL) spray bottle	STORAGE ADVICE
	Funnel	Refrigerate and use within 1 month

Honey

Who knew this classic sweetener was as good in your hair as it is in your cup of tea? A natural humectant, honey helps lock in moisture and prevents dry, brittle tresses. But its healing abilities go beyond hair:

Packed with antioxidants, this super ingredient is antibacterial, antifungal, and antiseptic, so it's also terrific at repairing and protecting skin. Here's how to get some of its sweetness into your everyday beauty routine.

EASY HONEY-COCONUT DEEP-CONDITIONING MASK

2 tablespoons coconut oil
1 tablespoon honey

Combine the coconut oil and honey in a small heat-safe glass bowl. Heat on the stove top or in the microwave until the mixture is warm enough to spread, then massage it into your scalp. (You can rub it farther down the hair shaft to heal split ends.) Cover with a shower cap for 30 minutes to 1 hour. Rinse and wash hair well.

BANANA-HONEY HAIR REPAIR

1 banana
1 tablespoon honey

Get double the moisture with these two nourishing ingredients. In a blender, combine the banana and honey, pulsing until all the banana pieces are well puréed and you've got a smooth mixture. Apply the mask to your hair, taking extra care to saturate the ends. Wearing a shower cap isn't necessary, but the heat it creates allows for extra penetration. Wait 20 minutes, then rinse and shampoo to remove the mask.

HONEY-YOGURT HAIR MASK

2 tablespoons organic, full-fat plain yogurt
1½ tablespoons honey
½ teaspoon coconut oil

Here, honey gets a helping hand from yogurt, which contains scalp-cleansing lactic acid and strand-strengthening proteins. Combine the yogurt, honey, and coconut oil in a small bowl and mix with a spoon. Massage the mixture into your scalp, working it down to your ends. Let sit for 15 minutes, then shampoo.

HONEY–OLIVE OIL TREATMENT FOR DAMAGED HAIR

½ cup (180 g) honey
¼ cup (60 mL) olive oil

While honey's humectant powers are great for hair, applying it to your hair gets sticky fast—try cutting it with olive oil for a less frustrating experience, and to coat and smooth the hair shaft. Mix the honey and olive oil together in a small bowl, then warm over the stove top or in the microwave for a few seconds. Apply from roots to ends and leave on for 10 to 20 minutes before shampooing.

Other Uses for Honey

BLACKBERRY-HONEY BODY SCRUB

Mash ⅔ cup (100 g) blackberries with a fork, or pulse in a blender until chopped. Add ¼ cup (90 g) honey and 2 teaspoons fine sugar; mix well. Use this body scrub all over—for optimal benefits, leave it on as a body mask for 10 minutes after scrubbing yourself down.

MOISTURIZING STRAWBERRY-HONEY FACE MASK

Mash 5 strawberries in a small bowl, then pour on 1 tablespoon honey. Mix together and apply the mask to your face, avoiding the eye area. Rinse after 15 minutes and follow with a moisturizer.

COCONUT-HONEY BATH MILK

Grind old-fashioned oats until you have ½ cup (50 g) powder, then combine with 1 cup (240 mL) coconut milk and 2 tablespoons honey. Add to a warm bath near you!

BUG BITE SOOTHER

Honey, the ultimate healer, can also soothe bites. Dab a tiny bit of honey on irritated areas to moisturize dry, itchy skin and take the sting out of the redness.

Rich Coconut-Pumpkin Mask

Your hair is really just protein—one called keratin, in fact. A great way to strengthen your strands is with more protein, so try this gelatin mask—which also gives a moisturizing boost, thanks to coconut milk and pumpkin.

1 / Measure and then combine the coconut milk and gelatin in a small saucepan. Heat the mixture over low heat, whisking until all the gelatin dissolves.

2 / Take the pan off the heat. Whisk in the honey and pumpkin purée—it's full of moisturizing vitamins, beta-carotene, potassium, and zinc. Let cool until lukewarm.

3 / Working with dry hair, apply the mask generously so that each tendril is saturated. Drape a towel around your shoulders to avoid drips.

4 / Wear the mask for 10 to 15 minutes. Don't let it dry or it will be hard to remove—this stuff is like cement!

5 / Rinse your hair thoroughly and follow with shampoo and conditioner.

MATERIALS	TOOLS	RECOMMENDED FOR
½ cup (120 mL) coconut milk	Measuring cups and spoons	Normal to dry hair
1 tablespoon gelatin	Small saucepan	
1 tablespoon honey	Whisk	FREQUENCY OF USE
2 tablespoons pumpkin purée	Towel	Weekly
		STORAGE ADVICE
		Use immediately

Triple-Threat Conditioner

This mask combines three natural-beauty mainstays for some serious deep conditioning. Coconut oil adds moisture and softness, argan oil helps control frizz, and shea butter remedies split ends and soothes dry scalps.

1 / Measure the coconut oil and shea butter. Combine them in a small heat-safe glass bowl, stirring to mix.

2 / Bring 2 inches (5 cm) of water to a boil in a small saucepan, then reduce the heat to low. Place the glass bowl inside the saucepan and melt the oils together.

3 / Remove the bowl from the heat, let cool for between 3 and 5 minutes, and add the argan oil. Stir to combine.

4 / Refrigerate the mixture until it starts to set (about 20 minutes). Whisk until it's frothy and easy to apply.

5 / Comb the mask through clean, dry hair and cover with a shower cap. Leave on for 30 minutes, then rinse your hair and shampoo as usual. Store any leftovers in a container with a lid, and enjoy again soon.

MATERIALS	TOOLS	RECOMMENDED FOR
2 tablespoons coconut oil	Measuring spoons	Dry hair
1 tablespoon shea butter	Small heat-safe glass bowl	
1 teaspoon argan oil	Spoon	FREQUENCY OF USE
	Small saucepan	1 to 2 times per month
	Whisk	
	Shower cap	STORAGE ADVICE
	2-ounce (60-mL) lidded container	Use within 3 months

Top-Knot Trick

A great general fix for extra-dry locks is to leave your masks on longer—just flip your head over, twist your hair into a bun, and secure with a clip. (For short hair, try a side twist.) Leave it up for 20 to 30 minutes—you can even go to the gym or run errands. When time is up, release the knot and hop in the shower to shampoo.

Get a Double Dose

You can easily double or triple the recipe for this ginger-infused hair oil. After straining out the ginger, transfer the oil to a jar with a lid. Twice a month, measure out the amount needed for your hair and warm before using. Just don't make it too hot—there's nothing beautiful about a burned scalp.

Citrus Shine Hair Smoothie

The next time you make a smoothie, whip one up for your hair too! In this recipe, orange juice enhances glossiness and pumps up volume, while bananas condition, yogurt adds protein, and honey locks in moisture.

1 / Measure and combine the orange juice, yogurt, banana, and honey in a blender or food processor.

2 / Blend until you've got a really creamy paste. Banana chunks are notoriously hard to remove from hair, so keep your finger on that blender button until the mixture has a supersmooth texture, like that of conditioner.

3 / Use your hands to slather the mask onto your dry hair. Don't be afraid to really pack it on, saturating the strands from roots to ends.

4 / Put on a shower cap to keep the mask in place and prevent drips, then grab a magazine and relax for about 15 minutes. Rinse thoroughly and follow with shampoo.

Tip / For extra volume, finish by rinsing with a can of strong ale (like Guinness). Let it sit for several minutes, massaging it into your roots, then rinse and style.

MATERIALS	TOOLS	FREQUENCY OF USE
½ cup (120 mL) orange juice	**Measuring cups and spoons**	**2 times per month**
¼ cup (60 g) organic, full-fat plain yogurt	**Blender or food processor**	STORAGE ADVICE
1 banana	**Shower cap**	**Use immediately**
1 tablespoon honey	RECOMMENDED FOR	
	All hair types	

Ginger Hot-Oil Treatment

Want hair worthy of a shampoo commercial? Mix olive oil (which delivers antioxidants and omega-3 fatty acids for extra luster) with scalp-stimulating ginger, then hit it with heat to help the nutrients penetrate the hair shaft.

1 / Grate the ginger root so you have ½ teaspoon, then combine with the olive oil in a heat-safe glass bowl. (Psst: You can substitute the freshly grated ginger with 1 to 2 drops ginger essential oil to simplify the process.)

2 / Bring 2 inches (5 cm) of water to a boil in a small saucepan and reduce the heat to low. Place the glass bowl inside the saucepan, simmer for 30 minutes, and remove the bowl from the heat.

3 / Strain out the ginger with cheesecloth. (In a pinch, a tea strainer also works well!) Let cool until it's lukewarm.

4 / To apply, work the oil into your scalp and then down to the ends of your hair. Comb through to saturate the strands. The longer your hair, the more oil you'll need.

5 / Wrap your hair with a warm, wet towel and sit for 20 to 30 minutes, then rinse and shampoo.

MATERIALS	TOOLS	RECOMMENDED FOR
1 small piece fresh ginger root	**Grater**	**All hair types**
3 to 5 tablespoons olive oil	**Measuring spoon**	FREQUENCY OF USE
	Small heat-safe glass bowl	**2 times per month**
	Small saucepan	STORAGE ADVICE
	Cheesecloth or a tea strainer	**Use immediately**
	Towel	

Color-Enhancing Hair Masks

The world's a colorful place—why not use its natural hues to amplify the tints in your hair? Herbs, fruits, and even veggies can bring out the highlights in blonde, brunette, and red tresses. Apply one of these masks twice a month, and you'll start to see the subtle changes add up. Sure beats a pricey trip to the salon!

BRUNETTE

1 / Bring the water to a boil in a small saucepan. Remove from heat.

2 / Drop in the black tea bags—over a few uses, this dark liquid will deepen and enrich your hair's natural coloration. Let steep for 5 minutes for an extra-strong brew, then let cool to room temperature.

3 / In a small bowl, combine ¼ cup (60 mL) tea with the cocoa powder and yogurt. Use a spoon to mix.

4 / To use, apply to dry hair and leave on for 30 minutes, enjoying the remaining tea while you wait. Rinse and follow with shampoo.

MATERIALS	TOOLS
1 cup (240 mL) water	Measuring cups and spoons
4 black tea bags	Small saucepan
3 tablespoons unsweetened cocoa powder	Small bowl
¼ cup (60 g) organic, full-fat plain yogurt	Spoon

RED

1 / In a small saucepan, boil the water, then take it off the burner.

2 / Add the hibiscus tea. Leave it to steep for 5 minutes, then let cool.

3 / In a blender or food processor, combine ½ cup (120 mL) tea with the strawberries—which teams up with the hibiscus to enrich red tints—and egg yolk for protein reinforcements. Pulse until mixed.

4 / Apply to dry hair and leave on for 30 minutes. Rinse and shampoo.

Tip / Even easier? Pour 1 cup (240 mL) cranberry juice over your head, sit for 5 minutes, and rinse.

MATERIALS	TOOLS
1 cup (240 mL) water	Small saucepan
4 hibiscus tea bags	Measuring cups
1 cup (125 g) strawberries	Blender or food processor
1 egg yolk	

BLONDE

1 / Peel and grate the potato. (While this gray tuber may seem an unlikely choice for a hair-color enhancer, the enzymes in the humble potato act as a natural lightener.) Use a cheesecloth to press and squeeze the juice from the gratings.

2 / Open the avocado with a knife and mash one half with the potato juice in a small bowl. Cut the lemon in half, juice one of the halves, and mix in the liquid using a spoon.

3 / To use, apply to dry hair and let it sit for 30 minutes. Then give your locks a good rinse and thorough cleaning with shampoo.

MATERIALS	TOOLS
1 potato	Knife
1 avocado	Grater
1 lemon	Cheesecloth
	Small bowl
	Spoon

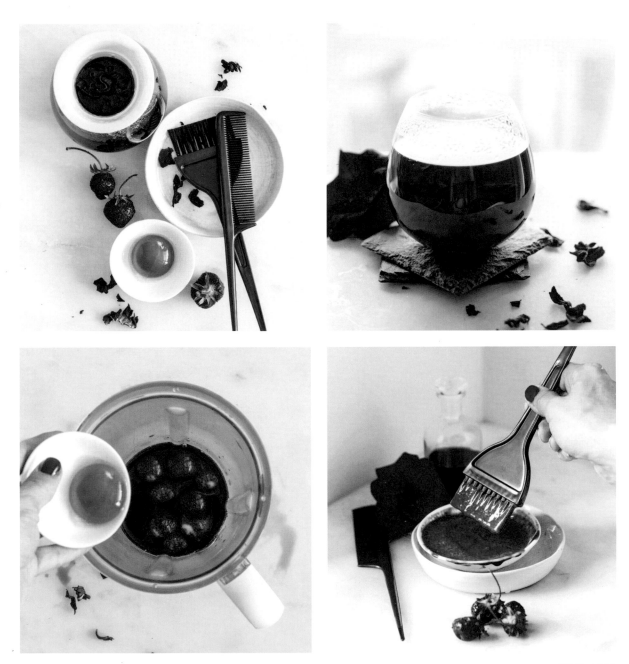

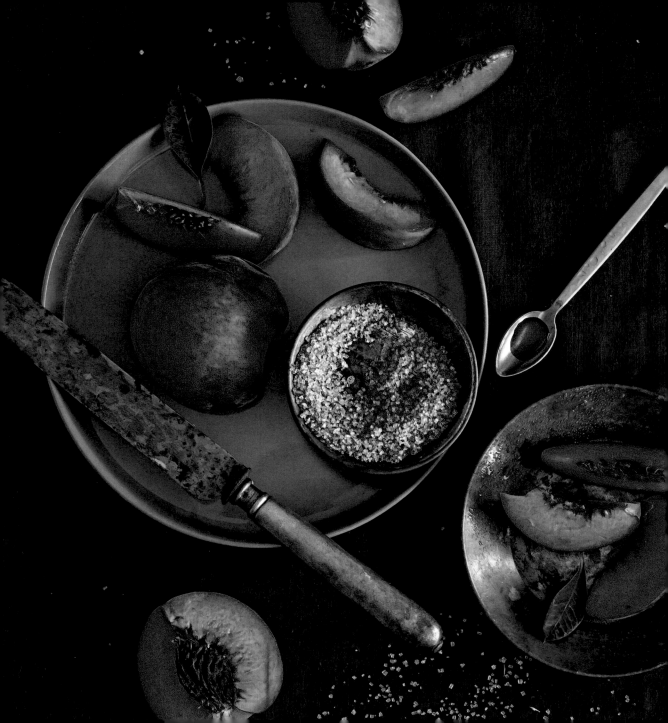

Nourishing Peach Scalp Scrub

Healthy hair starts with a healthy scalp. You can speed growth, halt hair loss, and stave off itches with follicle-declogging brown sugar and mineral- and vitamin-rich peach. Plus, who doesn't love a good scalp massage?

1 / Peel and pit the peach, then toss it in the food processor. Purée until you have a smooth consistency.

2 / Transfer the peach purée to a small bowl and stir in the brown sugar and jojoba oil with a spoon.

3 / Working with dry locks, apply the mask by lifting small sections of hair and slathering it onto the surrounding scalp. Massage thoroughly, using the pads of your fingers and even your nails to stimulate the scalp and increase circulation—it'll feel good!

4 / Leave the mask on for 10 to 15 minutes, then rinse and follow with shampoo and conditioner.

MATERIALS	TOOLS	FREQUENCY OF USE
1 peach	Knife	1 to 2 times per month
2 tablespoons brown sugar	Food processor	
1 teaspoon jojoba oil	Small bowl	STORAGE ADVICE
	Measuring spoons	Use immediately
	Spoon	
	RECOMMENDED FOR	
	All hair types	

Fenugreek Seed + Carrot Scalp Treatment

Merge the proteins and good fats found in these magic seeds with carrots' vitamins and silica, and you get a natural dandruff solution that also renews hair growth and strengthens hair follicles. Magic indeed!

1 / In a small bowl, combine the fenugreek seeds with the water. Let the seeds soak and soften overnight.

2 / Use a fine-mesh strainer to filter the seeds from the liquid, then combine the seeds with the carrot juice or purée in a food processor. (Why carrot? Its silica strengthens thinning hair and spurs growth.) Pulse until it's combined in a smooth paste.

3 / To use, apply the mask to dry hair, working in sections and paying special attention to your scalp.

4 / Let the mask sit for 30 minutes, then rinse thoroughly and shampoo and condition.

MATERIALS	TOOLS	FREQUENCY OF USE
2 tablespoons fenugreek seeds	Small bowl	2 times per month
½ cup (120 mL) water	Measuring cups and spoons	
¼ cup (60 mL) carrot juice or carrot purée	Fine-mesh strainer	STORAGE ADVICE
	Food processor	Use immediately
	RECOMMENDED FOR	
	Normal to oily hair	

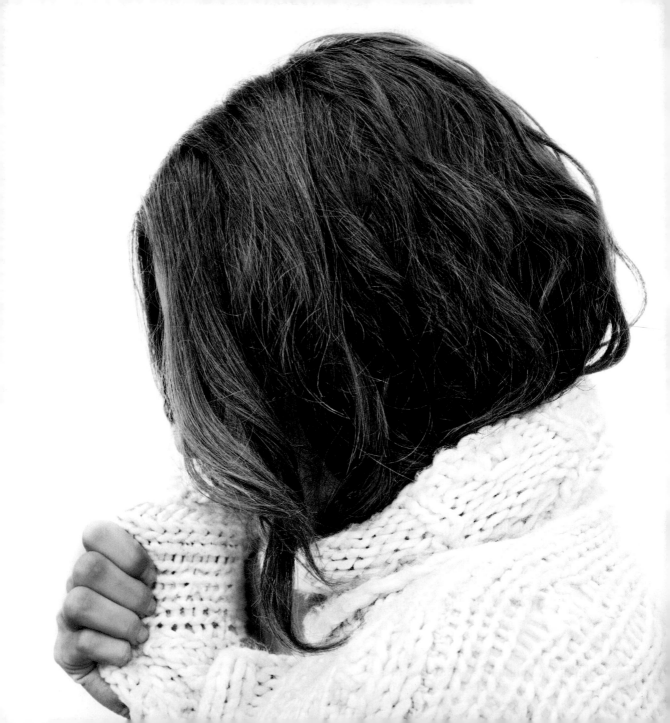

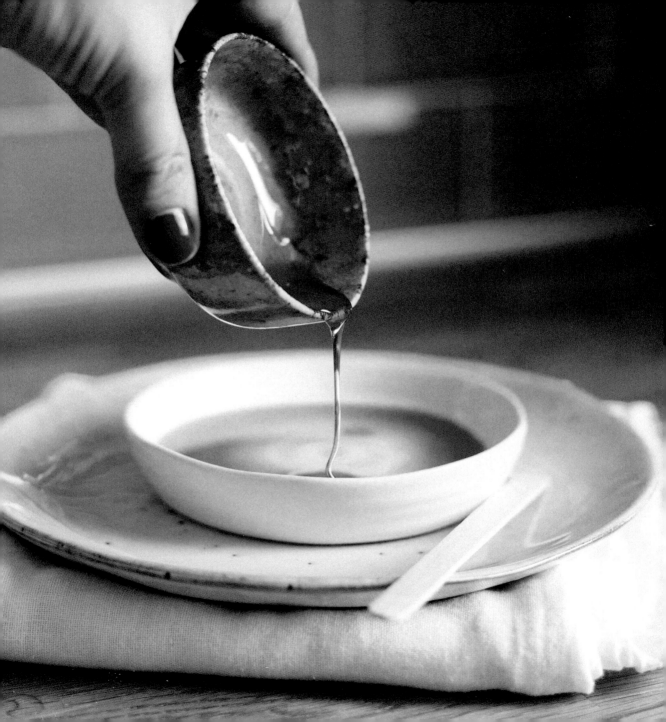

Avocado

One of the most popular "good fats," avocado is a superfood for both your diet and hair. Enjoy one in a meal daily (avocado toast, anyone?) and let its omega-3 fatty acids, vitamins, fiber, and magnesium nourish your hair and skin from the inside out. Then use a few once or twice a week in a natural beauty recipe to hydrate and protect from the outside too.

AVO-PEPPERMINT HAIR MASK

¼ avocado
3 drops peppermint essential oil

Use a fork to mash the avocado in a small bowl, then drizzle in the peppermint essential oil with a pipette. Wet your hair, squeeze out all the water, and apply the mask. Leave it on and relax for 15 minutes, then rinse and shampoo.

MIRACULOUS SPLIT-END SERUM

1 teaspoon avocado oil
2 to 3 drops rosemary essential oil

To minimize frizz, dispense the avocado oil into the palm of your hand. Use a pipette to add the rosemary oil, and rub your hands together. Apply to the ends of your hair (avoiding the scalp), comb through, and leave in all day.

AVOCADO-ALOE DE-FRIZZ SPRAY

1 teaspoon avocado oil
1 cup (240 mL) distilled water
2 tablespoons fresh aloe-vera gel
1 teaspoon glycerin

Mix the avocado oil, water, fresh aloe-vera gel, and glycerin together in a large measuring cup and pour into a spray bottle. Spritz on your hair to tame those pesky flyaways.

HIGH-GLOSS HAIR MASK

1 avocado
¼ cup (60 mL) olive oil
1 tablespoon lemon juice

Mash the avocado and mix with the olive oil in a small bowl—with their powers combined, the avocado and olive oil deliver major shine. Add in the lemon juice. Apply to your hair, leave on for 20 minutes, and then rinse.

COCONUT-AVOCADO HAIR SMOOTHIE

½ avocado
1 cup (240 mL) coconut milk
1 teaspoon avocado oil

Mash the avocado half, then combine it with the coconut milk and avocado oil in a small bowl and mix with a spoon. Massage the mask into your scalp and work it down to the ends of your hair. It's a good idea to put on a shower cap once the mask is applied: It creates heat, which helps the good stuff penetrate your locks more deeply. Let the mask sit for between 10 and 15 minutes, then shampoo.

Other Uses for Avocado

AFTER-SUN AVOCADO BODY MASK
Mash 1 avocado and mix it with 1 teaspoon honey and ¼ teaspoon lime juice in a small bowl. Apply the mixture liberally over the affected skin, then leave it on for 10 to 15 minutes to enjoy the full healing and hydrating effects.

AVOCADO ANTI-WRINKLE EYE TREATMENT
Scrape 1 teaspoon leftover pulp out of the avocado skin with a spoon. Apply it directly to your orbital rim (the socket area around your eye), then soak two cotton pads with cool water and layer them on top. Lie down for 10 to 15 minutes while this vitamin-rich part of the fruit hydrates your skin, then rinse with warm water.

DRY SKIN FACIAL SCRUB
Measure and combine 1 teaspoon fresh avocado, 2 tablespoons pulverized almonds, and 2 tablespoons coconut oil in a small bowl. Wash your face and apply the scrub to your still-damp skin with clean hands. Gently massage it into your skin for about 1 minute, starting with the jaw and working up. Rinse with lukewarm water.

Sunshine-in-a-Bottle Sea Mist

This sea spray gives hair loads of texture and volume—plus the smell instantly transports you to the beach! And if your hair is on the oily side, the salt naturally pulls out annoying extra moisture. Add in a small amount of oil to prevent overdrying, and top it off with lightening chamomile and lemon for those pretty sun streaks that tell the world you've been on vacation.

1 / Bring the water to a boil in a small saucepan. Remove it from the heat.

2 / Drop in the chamomile tea bag and let it steep for about 5 minutes. Discard the tea bag.

3 / Using a funnel, pour the Epsom and sea salts, almond oil, and tea into the spray bottle.

4 / Use a pipette to drizzle in the rosemary essential oil, then shake well so the salt is completely dissolved.

5 / Let the mixture cool inside the bottle. Stir in the fresh aloe-vera gel and lemon juice.

6 / Shake before each use and spray on clean, damp hair. Scrunch and twist with your hands to define the waves, then let your locks air-dry. You can spritz your look again once your hair has dried, if you're after a stronger hold.

Summer Haircare

All that heat, chlorine, and sea salt can really take a toll on your tresses. Here's how to keep the fun in the sun from frying your hair.

PRE- AND POST-SWIM Rinse with tap water and then spray in a simple detangling conditioner before diving in—it will seal the hair shaft and lock out chemicals. My go-to is 2 tablespoons all-natural conditioner, 2 tablespoons warm water per 1 cup (240 mL) conditioner, and 5 drops rosemary essential oil. Post-swim, rinse and spray your locks again.

GREEN HAIR MASK If you do end up with the dreaded green locks, mix ¼ cup (60 mL) lemon juice, 2 to 4 tablespoons baking soda, and 1 tablespoon liquid castile soap. Apply the mixture to wet, clean hair, massaging it in from roots to ends. Let it sit for 20 minutes, then rinse, wash, and condition.

SPF HAIR MIST You know it's important to protect your skin from the sun, but don't forget your hair! Dilute your favorite natural sunscreen with 2 tablespoons water per 1 cup (240 mL) sunscreen. Store in a spray bottle.

MATERIALS

1 cup (240 mL) water

1 chamomile tea bag

1 tablespoon Epsom salt

Pinch of sea salt

1 teaspoon sweet almond oil

4 to 5 drops rosemary essential oil

1 teaspoon fresh aloe-vera gel

1 teaspoon lemon juice

TOOLS

Measuring cups and spoons

Small saucepan

Funnel

8-ounce (240-mL) spray bottle

Pipette

RECOMMENDED FOR

Normal to oily hair

FREQUENCY OF USE

As needed

STORAGE ADVICE

Refrigerate and use within 3 months

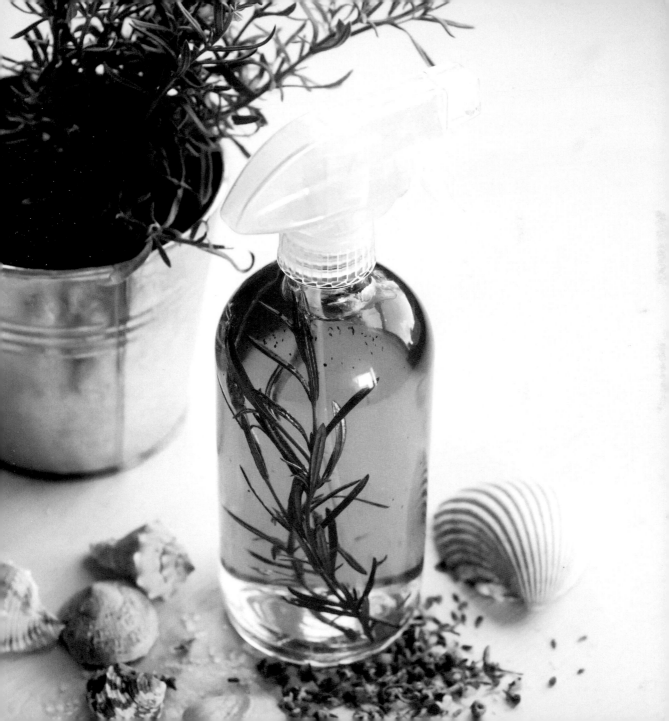

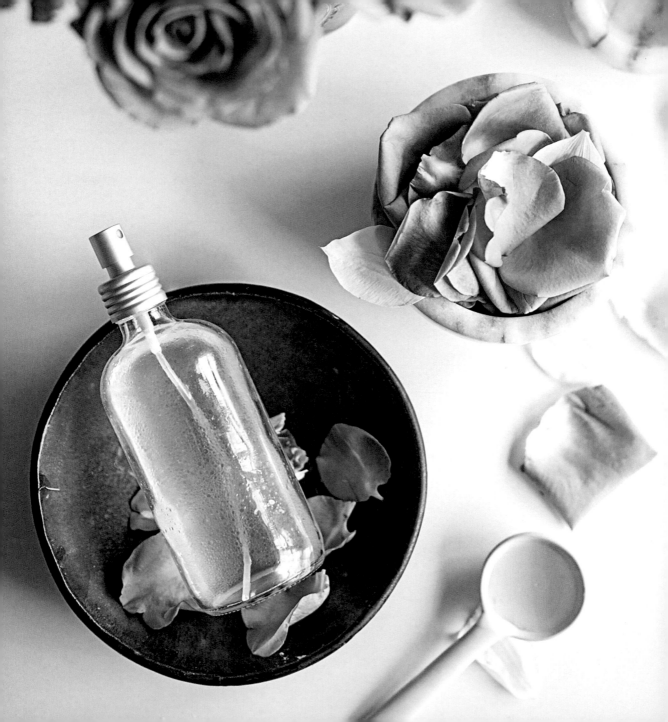

Rose-Water Anti-Frizz Spray

This homemade miracle worker harnesses soothing aloe, wonderfully scented rose water, and hydrating oils to add shine to frazzled locks. Use it on wet or dry hair to lightly condition and keep flyaways in check.

1 / Measure and use a spoon to mix the jojoba oil, glycerin, and fresh aloe-vera gel in a small bowl. (That aloe is crucial: It's a natural emollient that seals the cuticle and locks in moisture, preventing annoying frizz.) Whisk together until all the ingredients are well blended.

2 / Use a pipette to add the sandalwood essential oil, which adds a pleasant earthy scent and moisturizes ends.

3 / Pour the mixture into the spray bottle, add in the rose water, and replace the bottle's cap. Give it a shake.

4 / To use, spritz on wet or dry hair—it'll smooth down unruly frizz and hydrate the hair shaft. Be sure to agitate the bottle a bit before each use.

MATERIALS	TOOLS	RECOMMENDED FOR
1 teaspoon jojoba oil	Measuring cups and spoons	All hair types
1 teaspoon glycerin	Spoon	
2 tablespoons fresh aloe-vera gel	Small bowl	FREQUENCY OF USE
15 drops sandalwood essential oil	Whisk	As needed
½ cup (120 mL) rose water	Pipette	
	6-ounce (180-mL) spray bottle	STORAGE ADVICE
		Use within 3 months

Marshmallow Root+Argan Oil Detangler

If brushing your (or your child's) hair is torture, this spray will be a lifesaver. Boiled marshmallow root creates a slippery texture that makes tangles a thing of the past, while argan oil adds extra conditioning power.

1 / In a small saucepan, mix the dried marshmallow root with the water. Bring the mixture to a boil, then reduce the heat and simmer the herbs for 30 minutes.

2 / Remove the saucepan from the stove top and let it cool for several minutes. Using a fine-mesh strainer, filter out the herbs, collecting as much liquid as possible. Discard the solids.

3 / Let the liquid cool completely, then stir in the argan oil with a spoon. Transfer to a spray bottle.

4 / To use, give wet or dry hair a good blast with the detangling spray, then comb away those tear-inducing tangles. Shake well before each application.

MATERIALS	TOOLS	RECOMMENDED FOR
¼ cup (8 g) dried marshmallow root	Small saucepan	All hair types
1 cup (240 mL) distilled water	Measuring cups and spoons	
1 teaspoon argan oil	Fine-mesh strainer	FREQUENCY OF USE
	Spoon	As needed
	8-ounce (240-mL) spray bottle	
		STORAGE ADVICE
		Use within 3 months

All-Natural Vodka-Sugar Hairspray

I remember watching my grandma shellac her hair in an aerosol cloud when I was a kid. You can skip the fumes with this simple hairspray, which uses sugar to create awesome texture and incredible hold.

1 / Measure the water and sugar, and combine them in a small saucepan. Warm over medium heat, stirring with a spoon until the sugar has dissolved.

2 / Remove the saucepan from the heat and let the mixture cool down to room temperature.

3 / Add the vodka and stir together. Using a funnel, pour the mixture into your spray bottle.

4 / To use, mist your locks while they're still damp, then style as usual. You can spritz again after your hair dries to lock down your look.

Tip / Want more hold? Easy! Just increase the amount of sugar in the recipe to 1 tablespoon.

MATERIALS	TOOLS	RECOMMENDED FOR
1½ cups (360 mL) distilled water	Measuring cups and spoons	All hair types
2 teaspoons sugar	Small saucepan	**FREQUENCY OF USE**
1 tablespoon vodka	Spoon	As needed
	Funnel	**STORAGE ADVICE**
	12-ounce (350-mL) spray bottle	Use within 3 months

Balancing Cedarwood + Neem Oil Balm

Cedarwood and neem oils don't get a lotta love, but they're great in a healing hair balm. Naturally astringent cedarwood offsets oil, while antiseptic neem stops itches and flakes. Top it off with aloe vera to soothe and clarify.

1 / Combine the coconut and neem oils in a small bowl, and whisk until they're well combined. (If the coconut oil is solid, heat it up for a few seconds.)

2 / Pour in the fresh aloe-vera gel and use a pipette to transfer the cedarwood essential oil to your bowl. Whisk until the mixture is fully incorporated.

3 / Transfer the balm to a jar and let it sit uncovered for 1 to 2 hours. Replace the lid and store the balm in a cool, dry spot.

4 / To use, massage a small amount into your scalp. Leave the balm on for 15 minutes, rinse thoroughly, and follow with your shampoo and conditioner, if needed.

MATERIALS	TOOLS	FREQUENCY OF USE
2 tablespoons coconut oil	Measuring spoons	2 to 4 times per month
2 teaspoons neem oil	Small bowl	**STORAGE ADVICE**
1 tablespoon fresh aloe-vera gel	Whisk	Use within 3 months
10 drops cedarwood essential oil	Pipette	
	2-ounce (60-mL) lidded jar	
	RECOMMENDED FOR	
	All hair types	

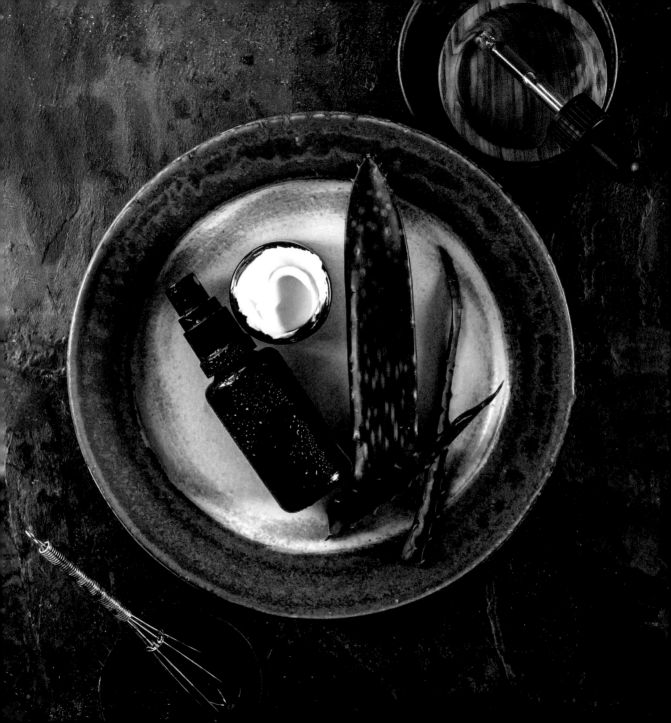

Eggs

Move over, frittatas: The good protein, fats, and nutrients in eggs can work wonders on your hair. If you have dry, damaged locks, egg yolks can rescue them with deep-conditioning and strengthening powers, as well as restore shine and volume. And instead of tossing those leftover egg whites, put them to good use tightening and firming skin (bye-bye, fine lines and wrinkles). Turns out having egg on your face isn't a bad thing at all—and that goes double for hair!

PROTEIN-RICH HAIR CONDITIONER

1 egg yolk
½ avocado

Separate the egg yolk from the white, then use a fork to mix the yolk with the avocado, which is excellent at smoothing out frizz. Apply the mixture to the ends of your hair—or massage it all over your head, if an all-over benefit is needed. Relax for 10 to 15 minutes. Rinse with cool water, shampoo, and rinse again.

MOISTURIZING LEMON–EGG YOLK MASK

2 egg yolks
1 tablespoon olive oil
¼ cup (60 mL) milk
Juice of 1 lemon slice

Crack two eggs and separate the yolks from the whites, then combine the yolks with the olive oil, milk, and lemon juice in a small bowl. Apply the mixture to your scalp and locks, then let sit for 30 minutes to allow the yolks to deliver their keratin-building protein and the milk and lemon juice to zap buildup. Rinse with cold water and follow with shampoo.

FRIZZ-FREE STRAWBERRY-EGG HAIR MASK

½ cup (60 g) strawberries
1 egg yolk
1 tablespoon olive oil

Mash the strawberries in a small bowl with a fork, then blend with the egg yolk and olive oil. Apply to your hair, focusing on the roots, and wrap your hair in cling plastic. Sit for 30 minutes to let the berries clarify and the olive oil hydrate, then rinse and shampoo.

EGG YOLK–HONEY SPLIT-ENDS HEALER

1 egg yolk
1 teaspoon honey

Separate the egg yolk from the white, and combine the yolk with the honey in a small bowl. Mix well with a spoon. Slather the mixture all over your hair, grab a good book or put on a movie, and then leave it on for 2 hours. (Yes, it's a long time, and, yes, it's worth it!) The honey in this luxurious treatment prevents dry, brittle hair, while the eggs' amino acids keep split ends from worsening. Finish with a rinse and a shampoo, and marvel at your hair's healthier ends.

Other Uses for Eggs

EGG WHITE FACE-LIFT MASK

Mix 1 egg white, 1 teaspoon lemon juice, and 1 teaspoon honey in a small bowl and apply the mixture to your face. Let the mask dry for 15 to 20 minutes, then rinse with warm water. The egg white will tighten and tone your face, while the lemon will reduce age spots. And the honey? It kills bacteria, as well as plumps up the skin.

BLACKHEAD-BUSTER MASK

In a non-metal bowl, beat 1 egg white until it's fluffy, then mix in ½ teaspoon clay and ¼ teaspoon lemon juice with a non-metal spoon. (Metal messes with clay's effectiveness, so use wood, plastic, or ceramic tools.) If it's a little too thick (which it may be, depending on your clay), add ½ teaspoon water. Apply the paste to your T-zone or blackhead-prone spots. Rinse with warm water after 10 minutes.

EGG YOLK HYDRATING MASK

In a small bowl, combine 1 egg yolk, 1 teaspoon olive oil, and 1 pinch turmeric to make a paste. Apply the mixture to your face and let it dry for 20 minutes. Rinse with warm water.

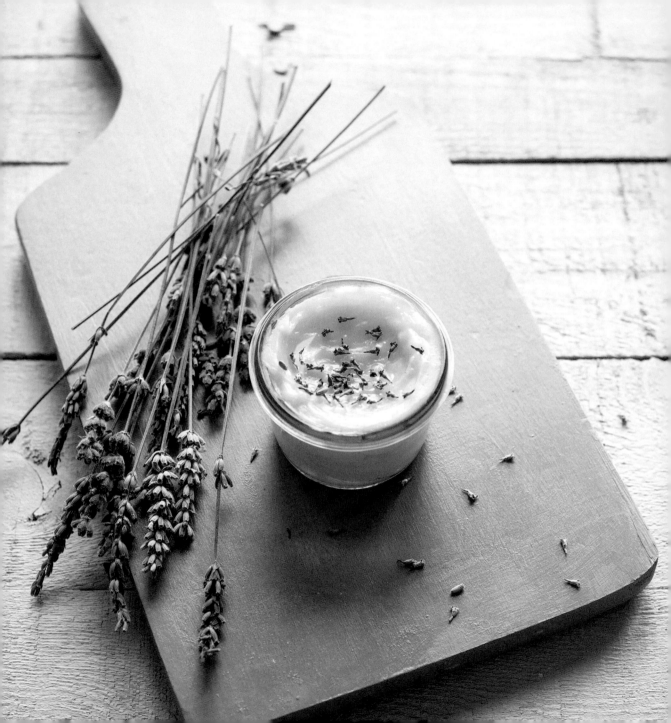

Lavender + Shea Butter Heel Balm

It's easy to ignore your feet, but they need just as much TLC as the rest of your skin, especially if you clock major hours standing or make poor footwear choices. Hydrate and heal your heels with this luxurious, rich balm full of ingredients that soothe and repair—including anti-inflammatory and deodorizing lavender.

1 / In a small heat-safe glass bowl, combine the beeswax, shea butter, coconut oil, and jojoba oil.

2 / Pour 2 inches (5 cm) of water into a small saucepan and bring it to a boil. Place the bowl over the saucepan and melt the ingredients over low heat, stirring frequently.

3 / Remove your mixture from the heat and let it cool for 1 minute.

4 / Add the lavender essential oil and stir gently while the mixture continues to cool.

5 / Pour the mixture into your jar and allow it to harden completely.

6 / Slather on this balm nightly before bed to relieve cracked or painful heels. Just be sure to put on socks afterward—unless you like greasy sheets. Use within 6 months.

MATERIALS

¼ cup (60 g) beeswax pellets

¼ cup (50 g) shea butter

¼ cup (50 g) coconut oil

¼ cup (60 mL) jojoba oil

50 drops lavender essential oil

TOOLS

8-ounce (240-mL) jar

Small heat-safe glass bowl

Small saucepan

Anti-Frizz Hair Spritz

From the frigid days of winter to summer's moisture-zapping sun, weather sure takes a toll on our tresses. Fight back with this hydrating spray, which contains aloe vera—to condition and nourish your hair—and jojoba and glycerin, which coat the hair strand's outer layer, smoothing the cuticle and reducing frizz.

1 / Whisk together the jojoba oil, vegetable glycerin, and aloe vera gel in a measuring cup with a spout.

2 / Drizzle in the lavender essential oil and stir to combine.

3 / Pour the mixture into your spray bottle. Be sure it has a good pump; if the nozzle is too small, it will get clogged easily.

4 / Fill the rest of the bottle with distilled water. For best results, refrigerate the bottle when not in use.

5 / To apply, shake well and spritz onto wet or dry hair from scalp to ends daily. Massage the mixture into your scalp, where the lavender will balance oil production and promote hair growth. Use within 3 months.

MATERIALS

1 teaspoon jojoba oil

1 teaspoon vegetable glycerin

2 tablespoons aloe vera gel

10 drops lavender essential oil

6 ounces (180 mL) distilled water

TOOLS

8-ounce (240-mL) spraybottle

Measuring cup

Whisk

Rainbow Dream Bath Bombs

No matter how chaotic life gets, you can always count on a warm bath! Beyond calming sore muscles and cramps, a bath is a great way to soak away a stressful day and turn a foul mood around. These bath bombs deliver the moisturizing goods (in the form of two lightweight oils) and a revitalizing, balancing blend of essential oils. Lemongrass cleanses emotional turmoil to promote confidence, while lavender, clary sage, and Roman chamomile ease anxiety and irritability.

1 / In a large bowl, combine the dry ingredients: the citric acid, baking soda, cornstarch, and Epsom salt. Stir to combine, breaking up any clumps.

2 / Combine the lemongrass, lavender, Roman chamomile, and clary sage essential oils with the sweet almond oil in a small measuring cup with a spout.

3 / Pour the essential oil mixture into the bowl of dry ingredients, then mix thoroughly. Divide the mixture into three smaller bowls.

4 / In the microwave, melt 1 tablespoon coconut oil in a spouted heat-safe glass measuring cup for 10 seconds. Continue with 5-second blasts until it's fully melted, stirring in between each.

5 / Add 2 drops of your first natural food coloring to the melted coconut oil. Pour the oil into one of the three bowls and use your hands to mix the contents together. Adjust the color, if desired.

6 / Repeat steps 4 and 5 with a different color. Repeat a third time so each bowl of dry ingredients has been thoroughly mixed with a different color of the oil mixture.

7 / Pack the mixtures into whatever mold you like, layering the colors on top of each other and along the sides of the mold. (If using a ball mold, as shown here, pack each side until overflowing, and squeeze both halves together to close.) This recipe will yield four bath bombs.

8 / Freeze for 20 minutes before use. To remove a bath bomb from the mold, warm the sides of the mold with your hands (this will help melt the coconut oil) and squeeze either side until the bomb pops out. Sprinkle with mica for a little shimmer, if desired.

9 / To use, fill your tub with warm water and drop in a bath bomb. It will fizz, releasing its scent and all its skin-softening agents. Soak for 20 to 30 minutes. Store in an airtight container and use within 6 months.

MATERIALS

½ cup (60 g) citric acid

1 cup (220 g) baking soda

½ cup (60 g) cornstarch

½ cup (120 g) Epsom salt

12 drops lemongrass essential oil

83 drops lavender essential oil

12 drops Roman chamomile essential oil

24 drops clary sage essential oil

1 teaspoon sweet almond oil

3 tablespoons coconut oil

Natural food coloring in 3 colors of your choosing

Mica (optional)

TOOLS

Mold

Large bowl

Measuring cup

Small bowls

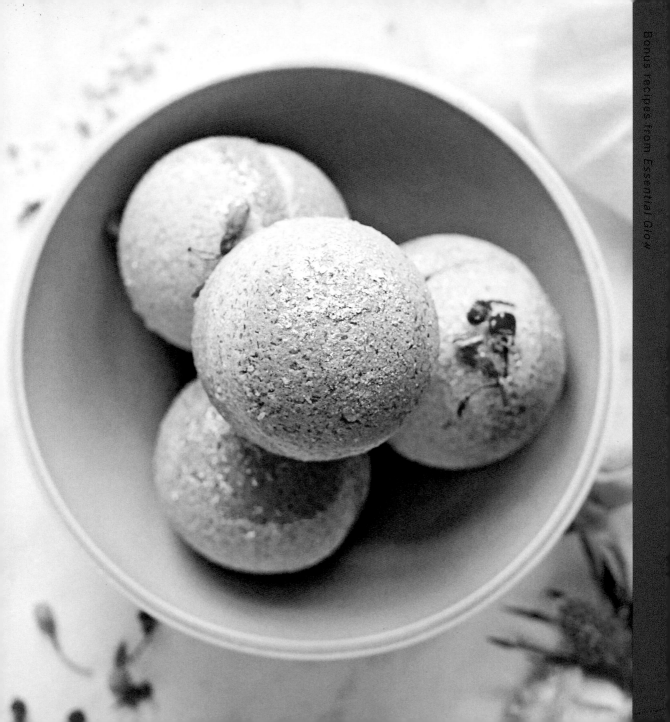

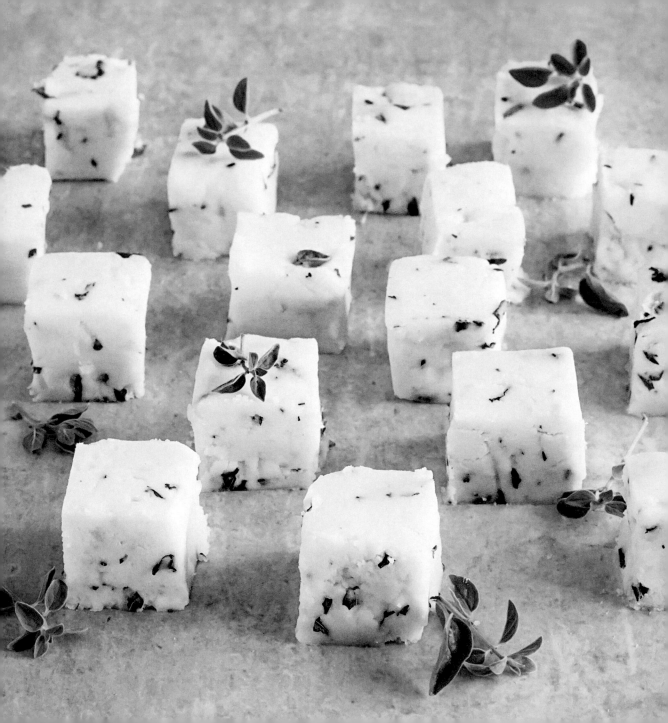

Herbal Facial Steam Tabs

I love a good steam session. It softens skin, increases circulation, and opens up pores so your favorite serums and moisturizers can penetrate the epidermis and do their thing even better. But a little tip from the esthetician: You don't have to visit the spa to enjoy the benefits of a good facial steam. These easy-to-make herbal tabs harness the antibacterial and anti-inflammatory benefits of oregano, which is used to treat both acne and rosacea.

1 / In a medium-size bowl, combine the citric acid, baking soda, and dried rosemary, thyme, and mint. Stir to combine, breaking up clumps.

2 / Decant the carrier oil of your choosing into a measuring cup, then drizzle in the oregano and eucalyptus essential oils.

3 / Pour the oil mixture into the dry ingredients, then stir until you arrive at a crumbly consistency.

4 / Use your hands to press the mixture into the wells of a mold. (A mini muffin tin or an ice cube tray works great for a batch of facial steam tabs.) Let them sit in a cool, dry place overnight.

5 / Remove the steam tabs from the mold and store them in an airtight container until you're ready to use them. (They will last up to 6 months.)

6 / When you're ready to steam, bring the water to a boil while you cleanse your face. Once boiling, transfer the water to a heat-safe bowl.

7 / Drop a steam tab into the bowl and immediately drape a towel over your head, shoulders, and the steaming water. (Or fill a sink with hot water, drop in the steam tab, and lean over the sink instead.)

8 / Keep your face about 12 to 18 inches (30–45 cm) from the steam. Enjoy for 5 to 10 minutes (and no more than 10!), then follow with a moisturizing mask or face oil. Keep your eyes closed to prevent irritation.

Tip / Oregano and eucalyptus are also great for stuffy noses and painful blocked sinuses. While your pores are soaking up the herbal benefits, take slow, deep breaths to bust up congestion.

MATERIALS

½ cup (60 g) citric acid

1 cup (220 g) baking soda

2 teaspoons dried rosemary

2 teaspoons dried thyme

2 teaspoons dried mint

2 tablespoons carrier oil, such as sweet almond or sunflower

10 drops oregano essential oil

5 drops eucalyptus essential oil

30-ounce (1-L) container

4 cups (945 mL) water

TOOLS

Mold

Medium bowl

Heat-safe bowl

Wipe-the-Day-Away Eye Makeup Remover

While natural cleansers are an upgrade over nonorganic versions, they don't remove mascara and eye makeup quite as well—and sleeping in that gunk can cause zits and even premature aging. This daily remedy goes easy on the eyes with witch hazel, jojoba oil, and aloe vera, plus lemon essential oil to cut grease.

1 / Combine the witch hazel, jojoba oil, and aloe vera gel in a small measuring cup. (Make sure your aloe vera gel is natural—not the goopy green gel you find in drugstores.)

2 / Pour the mixture into your bottle. Drizzle in the lemon essential oil, then replace the bottle's cap and swirl to mix the ingredients.

3 / Before each use, agitate the liquid to recombine. Then dispense a small amount onto a cotton pad, close your eyes, and gently wipe over the eye area. Don't tug or pull on the delicate eye area—it's a big no-no if you want to avoid wrinkles (and who doesn't?!). Be sure to use within 3 months, and avoid introducing water to the mixture.

MATERIALS	TOOLS
2 tablespoons witch hazel	3-ounce (90-mL) bottle
2 tablespoons jojoba oil	Measuring cup
1 tablespoon aloe vera gel	
2 drops lemon essential oil	

All-Natural Makeup Brush Cleaner

Think of your makeup brushes like paintbrushes: You wouldn't start a new masterpiece with dried-up pigment on your brushes—especially if you've invested in nice ones. Here's a simple, natural makeup brush cleaner that'll help keep your tools (and your pores) clear of old makeup gunk.

1 / Combine the liquid castile soap and olive oil in your bottle. (If it's a different size, adjust the volume—just keep the 2:1 soap-to-oil ratio.)

2 / Drizzle in the lemon essential oil, replace the lid, and swirl to combine.

3 / Before each use, first agitate the bottle to recombine the ingredients. Pour some of the makeup cleaner into a small dish. Dip your brush into the mixture and coat the bristles, then swish the brush back and forth in the palm of your hand. Get some good suds going!

4 / Rinse the brush until the water runs clean. Finish by spritzing it with a bottle of witch hazel to kill any bacteria. Lay the brushes flat to dry.

4 / Repeat as often as desired (after each use or daily, but at least weekly). Use within 1 year.

MATERIALS	TOOLS
¼ cup (60 mL) unscented liquid castile soap	3-ounce (90-mL) bottle
2 tablespoons olive oil	
5 drops lemon essential oil	
¼ cup (60 mL) witch hazel	

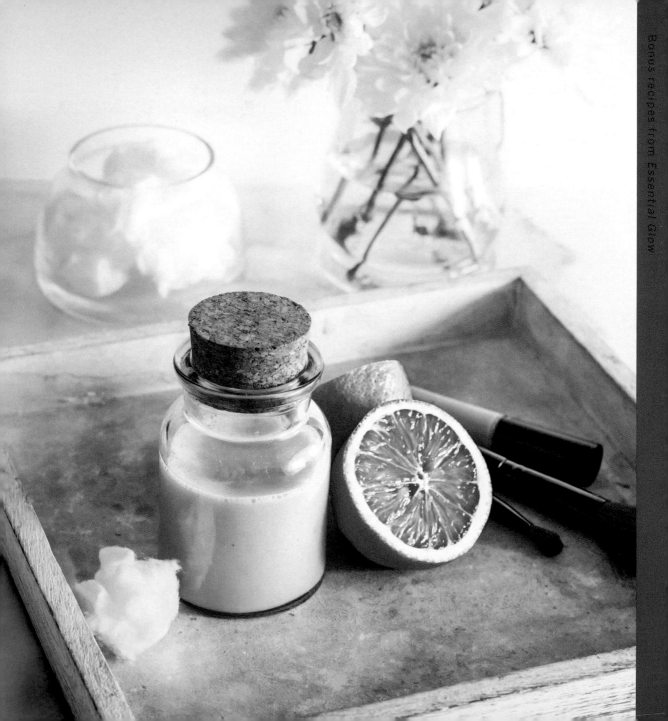

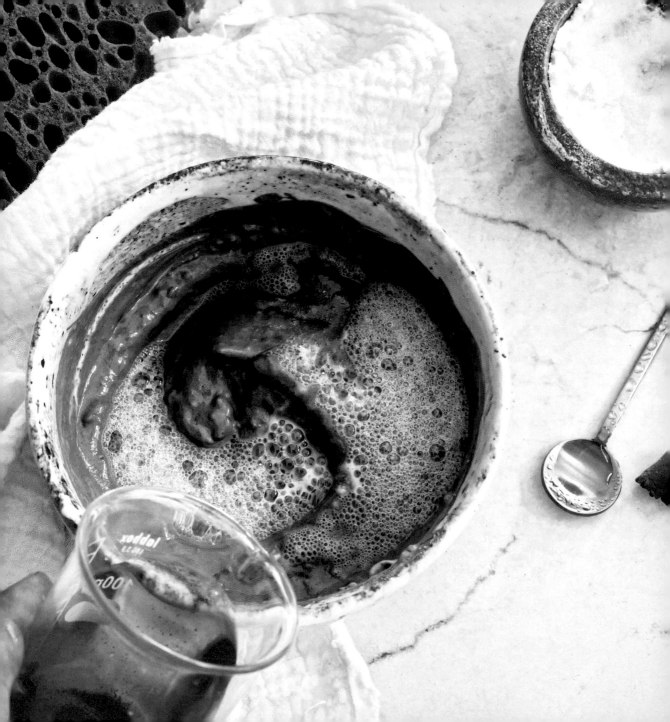

Carbonated Clay Mask

Carbonated clay masks have been a huge beauty trend, of late—and you can make your own without the cost. Instead of carbonic acid, this DIY carbonated bubble mask uses citric acid to get the same fizzy tingle.

1 / Combine the clay, baking soda, and citric acid in a small bowl.

2 / Stir until the ingredients are well combined.

3 / For extra detox power, you can add the activated charcoal or matcha powder now too, stirring again after adding.

4 / Pour in the glycerin and honey. Stir again.

5 / At the very last minute before you use the mask, add the rosewater and stir quickly. It's going to start to fizz, so you want to work fast!

6 / Use your fingers to apply the mask to your face and neck.

7 / Let sit for 5 minutes, then use a warm washcloth to gently massage the mask into skin. Rinse your face and pat dry.

Tip / Not only does this homemade bubble mask massage skin, but it helps remove excess oil and tighten pores, leaving you with a fresh, clean face.

MATERIALS

2 tablespoons rosewater

2 tablespoons bentonite clay

1 teaspoon baking soda

½ teaspoon citric acid

½ teaspoon glycerin

1 teaspoon raw honey

½ teaspoon activated charcoal or matcha powder (optional)

TOOLS

Small bowl

Calming Cucumber Mask

Winter air can leave skin dry and parched—but this calming and hydrating face mask will take the red right out of those windburned cheeks. Cucumber and oatmeal are both anti-inflammatory, sage is an antioxidant, and yogurt is one of the simplest and most effective face mask ingredients because it soothes and gently exfoliates.

1 / Puree a whole cucumber in a blender and measure out 2 tablespoons of ingredient.

2 / Add the cucumber to a bowl, and follow with yogurt, oatmeal, and finely chopped sage.

3 / Mix ingredients thoroughly. Note that the sage and oatmeal mean the texture of the mask will not be smooth, but they should still be evenly spread throughout.

4 / Massage the finished mask into clean, damp skin.

5 / Relax with this mask on for 15 minutes, then rinse to remove.

MATERIALS
2 tablespoons pureed cucumber
2 tablespoons plain yogurt
2 tablespoons oats, uncooked
1 teaspoon chopped, fresh sage

TOOLS
Blender
Small bowl

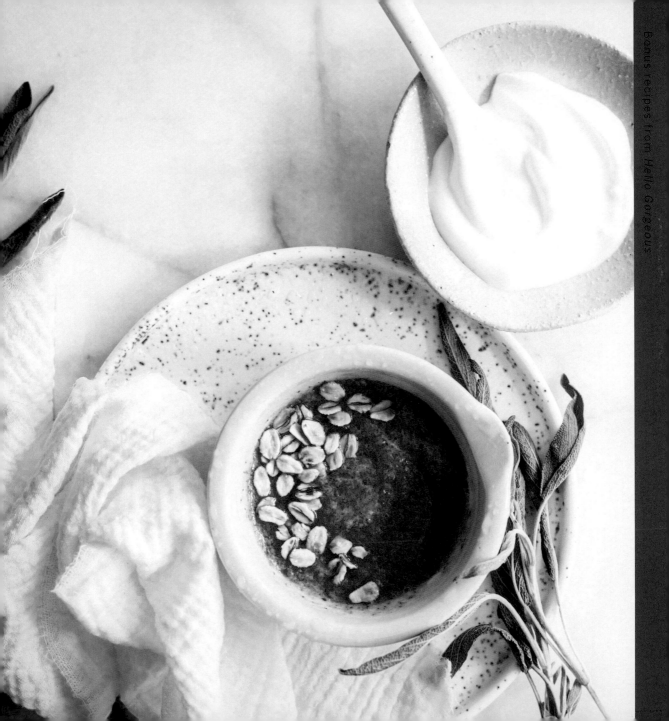

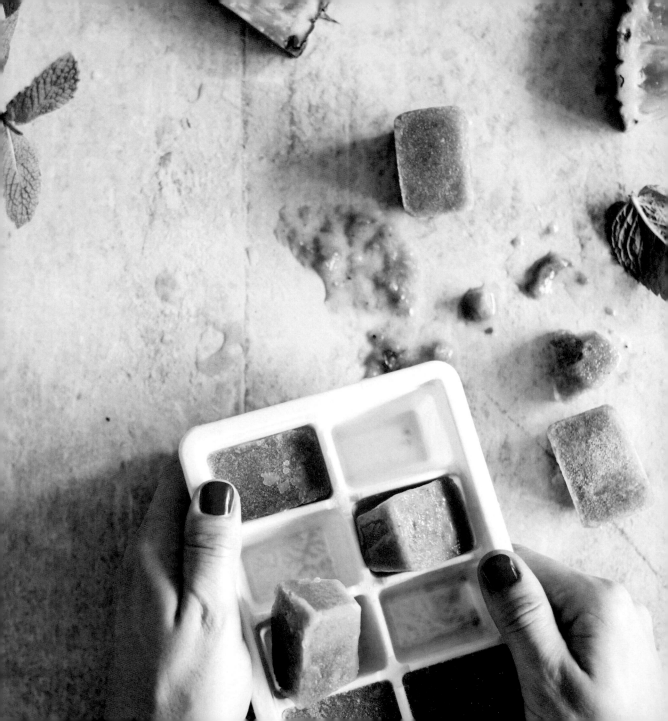

Tropical Enzyme Ice Mask

This tropical enzyme-packed mask is great for aging skin, pigmentation problems, and overall exfoliation. Packed full of potent vitamins and compounds, this mask will help dissolve dead skin cells while moisturizing ones that remain. It's a great mask for year-round use.

1 / Peel and seed the papaya.

2 / In a blender, combine all ingredients and blend until pureed.

3 / There is usually enough water in the fruit to let it puree well, but if you need to add a little water, go ahead.

4 / Apply some to your face immediately, avoiding the eye area, and pour into ice cube trays whatever does not get used immediately and freeze for a later date.

5 / Whenever you would like a mask, pop out a cube and defrost by placing in a bowl and leaving it on the counter until soft.

6 / You can mash the cube with a fork as it softens and then apply with fingertips, avoiding the eye area. Leave on for 10 minutes, then rinse with warm water and follow with moisturizer.

MATERIALS
½ fresh papaya, peeled and seeded
1 cup pineapple
5 strawberries
1 tablespoon honey

TOOLS
Blender
Ice cube tray

Dark Chocolate Honey Mask

Chocolate—just saying the word makes my mouth water. I love all things chocolate, from rich brownies and cakes to decadent truffles and nuts drenched in melted chocolate goodness.

Chocolate contains plentiful antioxidants that protect your skin and help reduce lines and wrinkles. But not all chocolate is created equal—for health and beauty, dark chocolate is the best.

1 / Add 2 to 3 inches of water to the small pot or saucepan and place the bowl on top, so that it's not touching the water.

2 / Heat the water to a simmer, then turn off the heat and add about half of the chocolate to the bowl and stir to melt.

3 / Stir in the remaining chocolate a little bit at a time, and mix until it's all melted.

4 / Remove the bowl from the pot and set on the counter to cool.

5 / Grind oatmeal in a coffee grinder, enough to get 2 teaspoons of ground oats.

6 / Pour the honey, yogurt, and ground oats, into the chocolate and mix the ingredients into a smooth, creamy paste.

7 / Massage the mask into your face with your fingers, using gentle, circular motions.

5 / Leave the mask on for 15 minutes, then rinse thoroughly with warm water.

Tip / Try to purchase chocolate with a high cacao content—at least 70 percent!

MATERIALS
3 to 5 squares dark chocolate
2 teaspoons ground oats
⅛ cup honey
1 tablespoon plain Greek yogurt

TOOLS
Small pot or saucepan
Heat-proof bowl
Coffee grinder

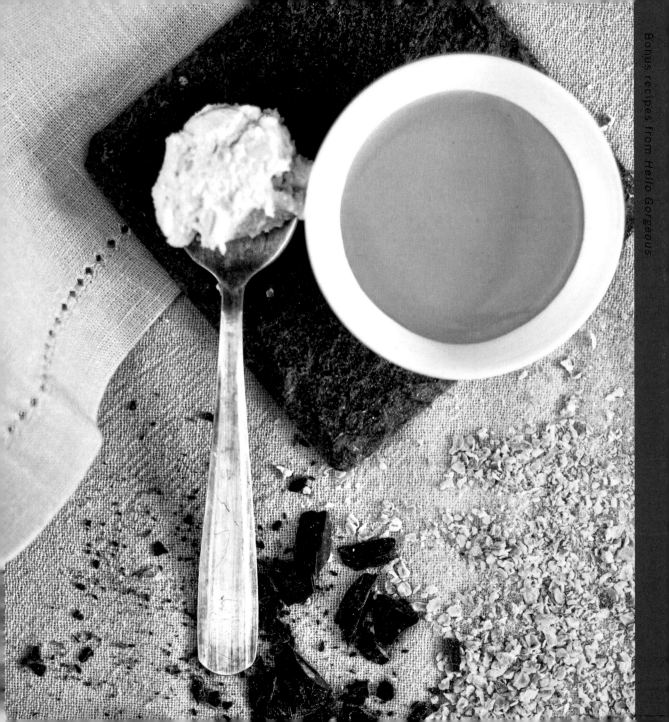

BEAUTY GLOSSARY

Acne When oil and dead skin cells clog up pores, it leads to inflammation of the skin glands and hair follicles—aka, pimples. Acne can strike at any age, so keep skin clear with regular, gentle exfoliation and treat flare-ups with herbs and essential oils that soothe inflammation.

Alpha Hydroxy Acid Forms of AHAs are go-to ingredients in many beauty and skincare products, especially anti-aging treatments. They exfoliate by breaking down the bonds that hold dead skin cells together and removing sun-damaged cells. There are several natural forms, including glycolic (found in sugarcane), malic (apples), lactic (milk and yogurt), tartaric (grapes and wine), and citric (lemon and grapefruit).

Antioxidant These are the good guys. They prevent other molecules from becoming oxidized and turning into free radicals, which can damage cells. Vitamins C and E are the most potent in fending off free radicals, so up your intake of superfoods like blueberries and green tea.

Astringent A common term that refers to a toner or lotion that contracts the skin. Witch hazel is one of the most commonly used astringents to tighten pores on the face or shrink blood vessels to relieve varicose vein pain. Lemongrass and mint tea are also effective astringents.

Blackhead The large pores on the chin, nose, and forehead are most likely to get clogged with dirt and oil, creating a blackhead on the surface of the skin. (Whiteheads are created by clogs under the skin.) To prevent, don't let makeup and other gunk sit on your skin overnight, and use regular clay masks to clear out and tighten pores.

Cellulite Short or tall, thin or curvy—cellulite is not selective when it comes to body type. Almost all of us suffer from dimples or lumps on our thighs, bottom, and abdomen as a result of subcutaneous fat deposits pushing up against other connective tissue. Applied topically, coffee is one of the best temporary fixes: The caffeine can tighten and tone tissue and help eliminate the toxin buildup.

Collagen A major building block of the epidermis, collagen is the protein responsible for skin's cohesion, elasticity, and regeneration. Upping your collagen intake via bone broth or supplements can greatly improve the look of your skin, help heal joint damage, and boost bone health.

Crow's Feet Yes, you can blame a lifetime of smiling for these fine lines that form around the outer eyes—but don't forget squinting and sun exposure too. Your best bet is avoiding sun exposure during the day (think SPF, sunglasses, and a hat) and slathering on a retinol treatment at night to reverse wrinkles.

Dandruff Your scalp can start flaking if it's dirty, dry, or oily. Other causes include sunburn, fungal infection, eczema, or sensitivity to a product you're using. Look for ingredients like tea-tree and neem oil, which heal and soothe the scalp.

Eczema This term can refer to a number of skin irritations that result in inflammation, dry skin, and a rash on various parts of the body. While you should talk to your doctor to determine the root cause, you can soothe the itch with witch hazel, honey, or a baking-soda bath. Avoid eczema triggers like fragrance, letting your skin get too dry, and too much stress.

Emollient Another term for moisturizer, an emollient keeps the outer layers of the skin soft and flexible, and provides a layer of protection to prevent moisture evaporation.

Exfoliation Run the back of your hand across your cheek. Does it feel dry or a little scaly? If so, it's time to exfoliate. Dead skin clogs pores and makes the top layers of skin dull and thick, creating unevenness in skin tones. There are two ways we can exfoliate: chemical and physical. Chemical exfoliation usually involves alpha hydroxy acids, while physical exfoliation uses small grains in a scrub to slough off the dead skin.

Free Radical When one of these unstable molecules attaches to a healthy skin cell, it causes a chain reaction of cellular damage and skin aging. Your body naturally produces some free radicals, but they can also invade the skin via pollution and other chemicals in our skincare products.

Humectant Some moisturizers, like honey, glycerin, and pulp from the aloe-vera plant, are categorized as humectants because they do double-duty for the skin, preventing moisture loss and drawing in more moisture.

Hyaluronic Acid A moisture-binding ingredient that supposedly carries 1,000 times its weight in water, hyaluronic acid often appears in anti-aging beauty products. (You can pick up an equally potent alternative in the health-food store: rose essential oil.)

Hyperpigmentation Dark splotches on the skin, often called hyperpigmentation, are usually the result of excess melanin, a pigment that creates skin color. Age spots are a type of hyperpigmentation caused by sun exposure. Tip: Try a mask with a little turmeric to brighten these areas.

Hypoallergenic This term is generally used to describe a product or treatment that's unlikely to cause a skin allergy or adverse reaction. Unfortunately, the term is unregulated in the cosmetics industry, so there's no common meaning for over-the-counter products. Buyer beware!

Omega-3 Fat These healthy fats found in nuts, seeds, fatty fish, and some oils are naturally anti-inflammatory. Plus, they boost epidermal moisture levels, keeping skin smooth and supple.

pH Scale This numeric system measures whether something is acidic (low in pH) or basic (high in pH). What does this mean for your skin? The thin, protective layer on the surface of the epidermis, known as the acid mantle, keeps moisture in and helps block out pollution and germs. To function at its best, it should be slightly acidic at 5.5 pH. If it's too basic (alkaline), skin can become dry and sensitive. A toner helps equalize the skin's pH after cleansing, bringing it back to its natural level.

Probiotic Doctors have long extolled the benefits of introducing these helpful microorganisms into the body. But these "live and active cultures" aren't just reducing inflammation and keeping your digestive system humming: Some dermatologists now advise probiotic supplements and a daily dose of yogurt to treat acne and rosacea. Further, Greek yogurt face masks may result in fewer acne outbreaks and better skin texture. Used topically, some strains of probiotics can kill the acne-causing bacteria hiding out in your pores.

Retinol Beauty aficionados are no stranger to seeing retinol listed on their product labels, especially those who buy anti-aging products. Retinol is actually the name for the whole vitamin A molecule, but it's artificially synthesized when used in cosmetics. It causes skin sensitivity and should only be worn at night. Frankincense essential oil is also an effective natural alternative.

Rosacea Most common in women over thirty, rosacea causes patches of red skin that look flushed or sunburned and often have visible blood vessels or small pimples. Rosacea isn't curable, but probiotic supplements and topical treatments of yogurt and/or aloe can soothe the redness and irritation.

Salicylic Acid A top ingredient in many exfoliating scrubs, this potent chemical removes dead skin and can help with acne. However, watch out, as it can also be very drying. Available over the counter, it's commonly prescribed mainly for its redness-reducing and pore-clearing properties.

INDEX

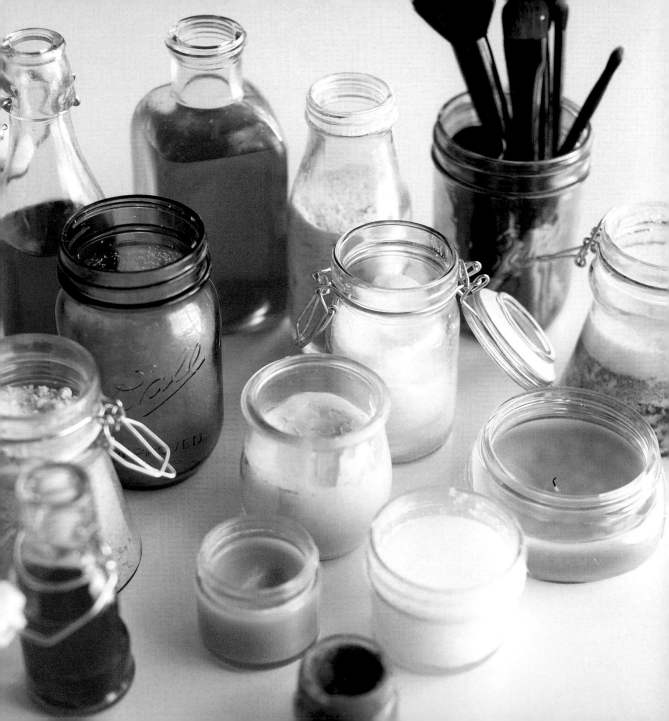

mists
  cucumber-peppermint face mist, 28
  sea mist, 138
moisturizers
  cuticle and hand moisturizer, 111
  geranium moisturizers, 37
  hibiscus bliss whipped moisturizer, 38
mud masks, 46
multimasking, 43

N

normal hair, 117

O

oats, 156–157
oil, 129
  balms, 24, 142
  detanglers, 141
  olive oil, 152–153
  treatments, 125
oily hair, 117
omega-3 fat, 163
oregano essential oil, 150–151

P

papaya, 158–159
perfumes, 108–109
pH scale, 163
pineapple, 158–159
probiotic, 163

R

rainbow dream bath bombs, 148–149
retinol, 163

rinses
  coffee hair rinse, 100–101
  green tea hair rinse, 45
  rosemary-nettle rinse, 123
roman chamomile essential oils, 148–149
rosacea, 163
rosemary, 28, 123, 150–151
rosewater, 154–155

S

sage, 156–157
salicylic acid, 163
scalp treatments, 33, 132. *See also* scrubs
scented oil, 108–109
scrubs
  blackberry-honey body scrub, 125
  cellulite-smoothing kiwi scrub, 89
  coconut-lime lip scrub, 66
  coffee cellulite scrubs, 100–101
  coffee-banana foot scrubs, 100–101
  dry skin facial scrub, 137
  mango scrub, 90–91
  mojito-mint foot scrubs, 104–105
  nourishing peach scalp scrub, 132
  tropical paradise mango scrub, 90–91
  whitening strawberry teeth scrub, 65
sea mist, 138
sensitive skin, 23
serums
  camu camu vitamin C serum, 37
  longer-lash serum, 59
shampoos
  customizable dry shampoo, 120
  tea-tree oil dandruff shampoo, 119
shaving cream, 111
shea butter heel balm, 146–147
shower gels, 98–99

skin peels, 33
smoothies, 52-53
soaps
  charcoal and tea tree oil detox soap, 93
  herb and spice glycerin soaps, 96–97
split ends, 145
spot remover, 106–107
strawberries, 41, 65, 125, 145, 158–159
sunburn soother, 33
sunscreens, 112–113
sweet almond oils, 148–149

T

tea tree oil, 93, 119
toners
  anti-aging green tea toner, 45
  balancing rosemary thyme toner, 28
  green tea facial toner, 33
toothpastes, 65, 111
thyme, 150–151
tropical enzyme ice mask, 158–159

W

wipes
  eye-makeup remover wipes, 62–63
  makeup remover wipes, 111
  rose and aloe vera face wipes, 30–31
  wipe-the-day-away eye makeup remover, 152
witch hazel, 152–153

Y

yogurt, 156–157, 160–161

weldon**owen**

an imprint of Insight Editions
P.O. Box 3088
San Rafael, CA 94912
www.weldonowen.com

CEO Raoul Goff
VP PUBLISHER Roger Shaw
EDITORIAL DIRECTOR Katie Killebrew
VP CREATIVE Chrissy Kwasnik
VP MANUFACTURING Alix Nicholaeff
SENIOR EDITOR Lucie Parker
ART DIRECTORS Lorraine Rath and
   Allister Fein
PRODUCTION MANAGER Sam Taylor

Copyright © 2022 Weldon Owen Inc.

Library of Congress Cataloging in Publication data is available.

ISBN-13: 978-1-68188-839-2

10 9 8 7 6 5 4 3 2 1
2025 2024 2023 2022

Printed and bound in Turkey.

Art Credits

ILLUSTRATION All illustrations by Masako Kubo.

PHOTOGRAPHY All photographs by Ana Maria Stanciu unless noted below.

Anais & Dax/AUGUST: 134 Laura Heller: 16 Susan Hudson: 49, 92, 109, 140, 149 Lindsey Johnson: 2, 4 (left), 5 (right), 79, 96, 99, 139, 146, 150 Stephanie Pollard: 149 Shutterstock: 9, 110–111, 144–145 Stocksy: 8, 19, 48, 83

Author Acknowledgments

Thank you to my sister, Susanna, for encouraging me to start blogging way back when. I think she was tired of hearing me ramble on and on about projects and recipes! And to my always supportive husband Mark, who never thought his English degree would be put to use reading beauty blog posts and draft after draft of facial recipes. Special shoutout to Pat, my invaluable kitchen assistant and recipe tester, who never wants to clean up melted beeswax again. And to my three special kiddos—Caroline, Henry, and Samuel—for inspiring this journey into natural ingredients and recipes.

Publisher Acknowledgments

Weldon Owen would like to thank Marisa Solís, Katharine Moore, and Kevin Broccoli and Laura Cheu of BIM Creatives for editorial assistance, and Deborah Harju for her professional esthetician consultation.

Disclaimer

The recipes, products, and advice presented in this book do not guarantee results and should not be used for treating a serious health problem or disease. If you have any concerns about your skin or hair, consult your personal health practitioner before applying any recipe from this book. If you have sensitive skin, always do a patch test for any new products or treatments. The author's testimonials in this book represent anecdotal experiences; individual experiences will vary. Neither the author nor the publisher may be held responsible for claims resulting from information in this book.